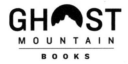

The
Doctor on Demand Diet

Melina B. Jampolis, MD

with Alice Lesch Kelly

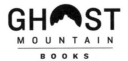

Medical Disclaimer

This publication is intended to provide helpful and informative material. It is not intended to diagnose, treat, cure, or prevent any medical, health, mental, physical, or psychological problem or condition, nor is it intended to replace the advice of a physician or other qualified professional. No action should be taken solely on the contents of this book. Always consult your physician or qualified health-care professional on any matters regarding your health and before adopting any suggestions in this book or drawing inferences from it. Health information changes rapidly. Therefore, some information within this book may be out of date, inaccurate, or erroneous.

Be sure to see your own health-care provider before starting the Doctor on Demand Diet or initiating an exercise program, especially if you have cardiovascular disease, diabetes, or any other health condition. The Doctor on Demand Diet is not designed for women who are pregnant or breastfeeding. Consult with your obstetrician, your baby's pediatrician, or other qualified health-care professionals on the best nutrition and exercise choices during pregnancy and lactation. This book may also contain suggested menu items. The inclusion of any menu items or references to any restaurants shall not be deemed, and are not intended in any way to be, an endorsement of the menu items or restaurants. The reader should always consult with the restaurant when ordering menu items.

The author and publisher specifically disclaim all responsibility for any liability, loss, or risk, personal or otherwise, that is incurred as a consequence, directly or indirectly, from the use or application of any contents of this book. Any and all product names referenced within this book are the trademarks of their respective owners. None of these owners have sponsored, authorized, endorsed, or approved this book in any way. Always read all information provided by the manufacturers' product labels before using their products. The author and publisher are not responsible for claims made by manufacturers. The statements made in this book have not been evaluated by the US Food and Drug Administration.

To Max and Beau,
for my daily dose of happiness.

Acknowledgments

First and foremost, I want to thank my patients for trusting me and allowing me to share in their weight-loss journeys. I learn something new every day from them, and that makes me a better physician.

Thanks to Alice Lesch Kelly, my cowriter, for being incredibly patient, understanding, and supportive throughout the writing of this book (which wasn't easy due to the fact that I was pregnant and then had a newborn!). Thanks also to Lisa Clark from Ghost Mountain Books not only for her helpful edits but also for her cheerful support (as a new mom herself!) and to the *Doctor on Demand* team for giving me the opportunity to write this book.

I also would like to express my gratitude to the following people:

- My friend and colleague Dr. Jennifer Warren, for being a wonderful cross-country sounding board and advisor throughout the writing of this book.

- Carly Stratton, for her cheerful enthusiasm and wonderful recipe-tasting feedback; Jon Ford, for his wonderfully thorough copyediting skills; and Ingrid Lopez, for helping me make many of the recipes during testing.

- Registered dietitians Jennifer Doll White and Jessica Ehrentraut, for their assistance; my fellow physician nutrition specialists Dr. Mike Rothkopf and Dr. Gerald Mullin, for their valued input; and my good friend Dr. Cindy Woods, for her reassurance and guidance.

- My pal, celebrity trainer Harley Pasternak, for his feedback on the interval training programs.

- Chef Michael Schley, for the tasty recipes that make this diet plan even better.

- Rebecca Raphael, for her editing insight, and my agent, Shannon Marven, for her continued support over the years.

- My friends Summer McKeivier, Brian San Marco, and Jennifer Herren, for helping brainstorm menus during playdates with our kids, and my wonderful sister-in-law Jordana Oberman, for helping so much with my newborn son when I was finishing up the manuscript.

- My sister Ami Jampolis, for always being a great sounding board and supporting me throughout my career.

- My amazing mother, Barbara, for her unconditional love and support on so many different levels, and my father, Sam, for being a great physician role model and always pushing me to excel.

- Finally, an extra big thank-you to my sweet and supportive husband, Benjamin, who did his best to keep me sane while I was going through a rough pregnancy and then giving birth while writing the book.

About the Author

Dr. Melina Jampolis is an internist and board-certified physician nutrition specialist (one of only several hundred practicing in the United States). Dr. Melina specializes exclusively in nutrition for weight loss, as well as disease prevention and treatment.

A graduate of Tufts University and Tufts University School of Medicine, she completed her residency in internal medicine at Santa Clara Valley Medical Center, a Stanford University teaching hospital. In 2005, Dr. Melina hosted a program on the Discovery Network's FitTV, *FitTV's Diet Doctor*, and for the past six years she has served as the diet and fitness expert for CNN Health.

She is currently the president of the National Board of Physician Nutrition Specialists and serves as the medical nutrition director for the advanced heart failure medical nutrition program for American Outcomes Management LLP.

Dr. Melina is the author of two previous books: *The No Time to Lose Diet* (in paperback as *The Busy Person's Guide to Permanent Weight Loss*), and (with Karen Ansel and Ami Jampolis) *The Calendar Diet: A Month by Month Guide to Losing Weight While Living Your Life*.

She believes wholeheartedly in the role of nutrition in preventing disease and achieving optimal health. Using balanced, sustainable eating, exercise, and behavior modification programs, she has helped thousands of clients over the past decade and a half to improve their health and well-being.

Dr. Melina is dedicated to the treatment and prevention of childhood obesity, particularly in the low-income, minority population. Her volunteer work includes helping to launch a healthy food pantry in the Hunters Point neighborhood of San Francisco, and biweekly family nutrition and obesity counseling sessions at the Los Angeles–based Bresee Foundation, a center for low-income, minority, at-risk youth.

She maintains a small private practice in Los Angeles, where she lives with her husband and two sons.

Contents

INTRODUCTION

—ɷ—

Weight Loss YOUR Way

During my years as a medical doctor specializing in weight loss and nutrition, one of the most important lessons I've learned from my patients is that one size does *not* fit all. People succeed at weight loss when they follow a diet plan that is customized specifically for *them*. The eating plan that works fantastically for a young parent may fail miserably for a busy executive; the recipes that satisfy a middle-aged man may leave a postmenopausal woman tired and moody; and the exercise program that galvanizes a couch potato may leave an athletic type feeling bored and uninspired.

My work with hundreds of patients has taught me that there is not a single "best" way to lose weight. But there are plenty of strategies that will work for *you*. The trick is to figure out what they are—and that's where I come in. My job as a board-certified physician nutrition specialist is to help patients improve their health and lose weight—not by following a one-size-fits-all plan, but by determining exactly what will work for them and their lifestyles. And as the author of the *The Doctor on Demand Diet*, my job is to show you how to create a just-for-you weight-loss program that can bring you a lifetime of success.

When I meet with patients one-on-one, I work with them to create custom-designed eating, exercise, and behavioral plans that help them meet their weight-loss goals. It's great doing this in person, but don't worry—you don't need weekly face-to-face doctor visits in order to succeed at weight loss. I'm not a psychologist, but I realize that there are often psychological issues that need to be addressed for any weight loss program to succeed long term (I discuss these in detail in Chapter 7). With the Doctor on Demand app, you can schedule a virtual visit any time with a Doctor

1

on Demand psychologist who can help you gain control over your eating behaviors, support your weight-loss efforts and provide you with even more tools to succeed. (And the Doctor on Demand physicians can even help you if you come down with a cold or flu or suffer a sports injury.)

I know the strategies, tools, and advice in the Doctor on Demand Diet work. That's because I interact on a daily basis with patients who are trying to lose weight, and I witness firsthand their struggles and successes. I understand that life is full of challenges, but I also have seen people overcome huge roadblocks that have prevented them from losing weight in the past. It all comes down to figuring out what will work best for *them*.

No matter what kind of life you lead, the Doctor on Demand Diet can bring you success. Whether you have a busy social life, a demanding job, a hectic household, or an erratic schedule, I can help you create a program that will work for *you*. Even if you hate to cook and have little time for exercise, you can still succeed at weight loss—provided your program is custom-tailored to *your* needs, *your* challenges, and *your* schedule, as it is with the Doctor on Demand Diet.

A Personalized Plan

Many factors contribute to weight-loss success. Your age, gender, size, activity level, health, and even your food preferences play a part. To be successful over time, a weight-loss program must take individual factors into consideration. That's exactly what the Doctor on Demand Diet does.

With the Doctor on Demand Diet, we'll start with a basic plan. Then, we'll work together—using quizzes, worksheets, checklists, and other interactive tools—to customize it to fit your goals, body type, personality, and preferences.

Along the way, we'll talk about more than just what you eat. In order to bring about long-term weight loss, we'll look at ways to make changes in behaviors that have contributed to excess weight gain. We'll also collaborate on creating an exercise plan that you can truly enjoy, fit into your schedule, and stick with for the rest of your life.

A Reality-Based Plan

In addition to being a physician nutrition specialist, I'm a mom with a very busy life. But I'm also someone who understands what it's like to always have to keep an eye on my weight. I'm not a naturally thin person, and in

Designed for You

Your own Doctor on Demand Diet plan will focus on your needs, goals, and choices. For example:

- *If you're in a hurry to see results,* I'll show you how to customize a plan that will bring about accelerated weight loss. But if you're more of a tortoise than a hare, we'll work together to design a slower-but-steady approach.

- *If you are insulin-resistant,* we'll design an eating plan that focuses specifically on stabilizing blood sugar levels. (Insulin resistance is a condition in which your body doesn't use insulin effectively to deliver blood sugar to your cells—I'll explain it in detail later in the book.) Everyone can benefit from blood sugar stabilization, so it's an important part of any weight-loss plan. I'll help you determine your insulin status, and together we'll design a program that best supports your health.

- *If feeling hungry is a major challenge for you,* you can create meals and snacks for optimal fullness and satiety.

- *If you like to splurge a bit on weekends,* you can use my Diet-Cycling strategies to enjoy wine, desserts, or other treats on the weekends without setting yourself back and regaining weight.

my teens and 20s—in high school, college, and medical school—I sometimes struggled with my weight. Over the years I figured out what works for me, and these days I do a pretty good job of keeping my weight in the right place. But it's something I always have to watch—if I'm not mindful of what I eat and how much I exercise, my weight starts inching up. And like many other women, I've faced the challenge of losing pregnancy weight after the births of each of my children.

Because maintaining a healthy weight is a personal commitment as well as a professional passion, I promise you that, above all, the Doctor on Demand Diet is realistic. I don't ask you to make huge, dramatic changes in your diet or to give up entire food groups for the rest of your life—unless of course you are a total junk food junkie, in which case I will definitely nudge you to make some big changes. But I don't expect you to follow ridiculous advice that I couldn't adhere to myself—in fact, I put all my recommendations to the "Could I do it?" test, and if the answer is "Absolutely not!" I don't suggest them.

And I don't expect you to make every change I recommend. You don't have to be a trained seal following a long list of orders. Successful weight loss is not about me telling you what to do—it's about us working together to build a program that will be just right for you and the life you lead. Some of my strategies will work well for you; others may send you running in the other direction. That's fine—this plan is all about customization. My job is to give you lots of options; your job is to use the information and concepts in this book to find the best approach for you, and to stick with that approach most (but not all) of the time.

You *can* lose weight. Even if you've tried and failed many times before, you can succeed at shedding excess pounds that weigh down your spirit and your health. All you need is a plan that really, truly works *for you*, one that is built around *your life* and that understands *your needs*. In the pages that follow, I'll work with you to devise your perfect weight-loss program. I'll be with you, every step of the way—as will the Doctor on Demand app if you need a little extra advice or support to succeed.

Highlights of the Doctor on Demand Diet

The Doctor on Demand Diet is not like other weight-loss plans. It is a flexible, customizable, reality-based program that meets you where you are now and leads you through a series of steps that allow you to personalize your own best weight-loss game plan. I'll explain the Doctor on Demand Diet in detail as we go along, but for now, here are some of the highlights you can look forward to:

A Truly Realistic, Personalized Eating Plan

The Doctor on Demand Diet builds on everyday foods that *you* already eat—there's no need to throw out everything in your kitchen and replace all of your favorite foods with expensive, unfamiliar substitutes, as some diet books recommend. Sure, I'll be suggesting that you occasionally try a nutritious new food or recipe, and if you like it, you can add it to your repertoire. But overall, you'll be focusing on foods that you already enjoy and can buy in your local grocery store—no need to run from one expensive store to the next for hard-to-find ingredients and overpriced specialty items.

Strategies Customized for You

I don't believe in one-size-fits-all recommendations for calories, protein, carbohydrates, or fat. For example, a middle-aged five-foot-two woman has very different dietary needs than a young six-foot-two man. An obese person needs a different approach than someone who's just trying to go down a dress size. A physically active person can eat more than someone who does no exercise—although I encourage everyone to be as active as they are able.

With the Doctor on Demand Diet, I'll show you how to customize your eating plan based on a range of factors, including how much weight you want to lose, how much you like to cook, what foods you like to eat, and what kind of life you lead. You'll know exactly how much of each kind of food *you* should eat to achieve the weight loss you desire.

Tried-and-True Advice from My Clinical Practice

Many popular diet books are written by celebrities, trainers, and sometimes just people who have succeeded at losing weight. Few of these "experts" interact directly with real people who are struggling with weight loss on a daily basis. But I do. As a physician nutrition specialist, I help people just like you to lose weight, not with the use of pills and surgery, but through behavior and nutritional changes.

All of my patients are trying to lose weight, and in the process of working with them for many years, I have learned a lot about how to succeed at it. The suggestions, strategies, and tips in this book are based on my clinical experience with all kinds of patients. When I offer advice, you can be sure it's the real deal.

A Program Built on Science

I'm a physician, so my first priority is always to give patients a weight-loss program that makes their health a top priority. That's why the Doctor on Demand Diet is based on the science of smart weight loss. It's not a crazy fad diet that slashes calories by asking you to eliminate entire food groups.

Yes, I'll ask you to make some short-term sacrifices—for example, I'll make a case for avoiding several kinds of "dry carbohydrates" during your first 10 days of the plan. (Dry carbs are breads, crackers, waffles, certain snacks, and other foods that are made with refined carbohydrates and that do a poor job of satiating hunger—I'll explain more about them later.) But after that, you'll use a variety of research-based strategies to incorporate all kinds of foods into your weight-loss plan, which will allow you to lose weight while improving your overall health. And you'll learn some simple, easy-to-schedule strategies to make fitness activities a permanent part of your life.

Quizzes and Questionnaires That Pinpoint Your Needs

When I meet with patients one-on-one, I spend a lot of time asking questions about what they like to eat, when they're hungriest, which foods fill them up, and how their moods are impacted by food, to name just a few. We use the answers to those kinds of questions to customize patients' weight-loss plans.

In the Doctor on Demand Diet, we use quizzes, questionnaires, and other tools to gather information that will allow you to personalize a plan that best fits your personal weight-loss style. For example, one of my quizzes will help you determine whether you are engaging in binge eating. Another quiz will help you understand what kind of exerciser you are, so you can choose activities that groove with your personal fitness style. Using the results of these tools, you can customize a plan that will be tailor-made for you.

Inspiring, Informative "SOAP Notes" from My Practice

These sound like something from a bubble bath, but they're actually an incredibly beneficial tool that will help you design your Doctor on Demand eating plan so that it will meet your specific needs. SOAP stands for Subjective, Objective, Assessment, and Plan, and a SOAP Note is a tool that all physicians and other health-care providers use to document information in a patient's record.

After meeting a patient each week, I write SOAP Notes that delineate the patient's successes, challenges, achievements, and goals, as well as the specific tips, strategies, and advice that helped or hindered them since the last visit. In the pages that follow I'll share some of my most compelling SOAP Notes (with my patients' privacy and identities fully protected, of course). The patients whose SOAP Notes I share are real people just like you—people with busy schedules who don't have time to make weight loss a full-time job. They represent a very diverse group of individuals, with equally diverse eating, exercise, and behavioral issues. Reading about the various ways my patients and I worked together to personalize their diets, behavior choices, and exercise programs will inspire you, and it will help us devise strategies that work for you.

Worksheets That Work

My patients love to use interactive worksheets like the ones I include in this book to better understand what drives their eating behaviors. Filling them out will help you identify challenges, brainstorm solutions, recognize successes, and pinpoint strategies that work and don't work for you. They'll also come in handy if you choose to connect with a health-care provider through the Doctor on Demand app.

Enlightening "Research on Demand" Summaries

Because weight loss and dietary health are so crucial, researchers around the world are devoting an amazing amount of time and energy to the study of optimizing nutrition and losing weight. The findings from some of these studies can often provide really helpful insights that can guide us as we create winning weight-loss plans.

Don't worry: I'm not going to ask you to pore over medical journals—that's a fun way for me as a doctor to pass an evening, but I don't expect it of you. Instead, I'll include quick, easy-to-read Research on Demand summaries that will keep you abreast of some of the exciting findings in the world of weight-loss research. Just look for the Research on Demand icon. And for those who want to find out more about the studies, I'll provide links to the original research abstracts in the bibliography at the end of the book.

No-Cook, Low-Cook, and Slow-Cook Recipes

I always laugh when I hear about diets that required hours at the stove every day. Sure, some people have the time and the interest to cook elaborate meals. But in my experience—personally and professionally—recipes with dozens of ingredients and long cooking times just don't fit into most people's lives. That's why most of the Doctor on Demand recipes are quick and easy.

If you, like me, barely have the knowledge or energy to boil water, you'll love having a choice of recipes that respect your time and interest level (or lack thereof). Whenever possible, I've included quick-fix, time-saving options. Many of the recipes I include in this book require little or no cooking. So if you're not an in-the-kitchen gal or guy, you'll have plenty of options that fit your lifestyle. And most of my slow-cook and soup recipes freeze well, so when you're in the mood you can cook them up and put them away for busy-day meals. Plus, I'll show you lots of ways to incorporate super-nutritious foods, such as beans and greens—two of my nutrient-rich favorites—into quick-prep meals and snacks.

The recipes in the Doctor on Demand Diet come from one of my favorite chefs. Michael Schley is a professional chef with lots of amazing experience, including a stint at one of the top restaurants in Northern California. He's also a member of my family, so he totally understands my work and my patients' needs. Working closely with me, Michael has created many recipes that are not only easy to make in most cases, but fantastically delicious. I've also created a few that are even simpler but equally tasty. These recipes are so good that you'll want to make them a permanent part of your recipe repertoire for years to come. When your goal is long-term success, you need recipes that will stand the test of time.

On Demand Meal "Templates"

Chef Michael and I have also created a selection of On Demand meal templates that you can use for a lifetime of healthy meals. Meal templates start with structured recipes, but then we mix in a big measure of flexibility, giving you countless ways to customize your meals by choosing which proteins, vegetables, spices, grains, fruits, and flavors you like most.

For example, the On Demand stir-fry template will show you how to make many different stir-fries rather than just one. And with the On Demand smoothie template, you'll be on your way to making dozens of different smoothies by altering the fruit, protein, and other add-ins you choose to use.

Clinical Pearls: *Tips That Really Work*

In medicine we have something called "clinical pearls," which are practice-based tips and advice. When I come across an idea or tip that is really helpful—something that my patients have found works really well—I'll share it with you. Just look for the Clinical Pearl icon. ◇

Reality-Based Exercise Strategies

Exercise is a crucial part of successful weight loss. But I know you probably don't have time to spend hours every day in the gym. So I focus on easy ways to incorporate activity into your day. For example, exercise scientists have identified a neat way to burn extra calories—and by "neat" I mean NEAT, which stands for non-exercise activity thermogenesis. Using the principles of NEAT, I'll show you some, yes, neat ways to increase your fitness level and burn extra calories simply by adding tiny bouts of activity to your day—we're talking about just a few minutes here and a few minutes there. I'll also tell you about interval training, which gives you a fantastic bang for your exercise buck—it's the fastest, most schedule-savvy way to work exercise into your life.

A "Structured Flexibility" Approach

When it comes to successful weight loss, I've found that people need two things: structure and flexibility. That may sound counterintuitive, since structure and flexibility seem to be polar opposites. But combining them into a "structured-flexibility" approach actually makes a lot of sense.

Here's why: People who are setting out to lose weight want to know what they ought to eat. Once they figure that out, though, they need to know how they can be flexible enough to work around the challenges posed by their schedules, personal preferences, and other issues that they face every day. That requires a careful mix of structure and flexibility, which is one of the best parts of the Doctor on Demand Diet.

Here's an example of how my structured-flexibility approach works: Although I'll recommend that you cut back on sweets (structure), I'm not going to tell you to eliminate every single gram of sugar from your diet (flexibility). Instead, I'll help you figure out how to find a balance that allows you to lose weight without losing your mind.

For example, if you find unflavored nonfat Greek yogurt a little too plain for your liking, we'll talk about whether it makes sense to use a bit of honey, sugar, or no-calorie sweetener to make this super-healthy food more palatable. And if occasionally giving in to a craving is a strategy that works for you, then I'll give you permission to embrace it! It's all about understanding exactly what works for you.

Our goal is not to have the top spot on the Perfect Diet Honor Roll. It's to get you to a better place physically and emotionally by improving your diet and boosting your overall health—and in my experience, structured flexibility serves you far more effectively than rigidity.

A Long-Term Resource

Although the recommendations in this book can deliver exciting results, the Doctor on Demand Diet is definitely not a quick-fix fad plan. Rather, it is a permanent weight-loss resource that you can rely on today, tomorrow, and for the rest of your life. By following the strategies, recommendations, and recipes in this book, you can lose excess weight and keep it off.

Now that you know what to expect from the Doctor on Demand Diet, let's get going!

A Strong Foundation

—✳—

Before You Get Started

Before you begin following the Doctor on Demand Diet, there are four things you can do that will dramatically boost your chances of success:

1. Start keeping a food and exercise journal.

Research has found that the very simple act of writing down what you eat can help bring about weight loss. In fact, in some studies, keeping a food journal is the top predictor of long-term success. This is something I've seen with my patients—when they keep track of what they eat, they are more likely to stick with their weight-loss plan and see great results than those who don't.

To help you with this, I've created a sample food and exercise journal page at the end of chapter 1. You can also use a notebook, an online spreadsheet, a food journal app, your daily planner, or even the notes section on your smartphone—it doesn't matter how you do it, as long as you make note of what, when, and how much you eat. (I also provide an exercise-only journal template page in chapter 6 for people who prefer to track their exercise separately.)

In your food journal you can also include notes that will guide you as you customize your personal weight-loss plan. For example, if you're particularly hungry one day, or if you find that a certain meal is especially satisfying (or not), make a note of it. This will help you to tailor your personal plan going forward. Many people also find that recording their mood or location helps them identify problem situations. A food journal can really help you pinpoint times or places that you may be eating more than you realize, or where you could cut back a little.

I've found keeping a food journal really helps my patients stay on track. In fact, I use a food journal myself! You won't have to keep using it forever (unless you want to), but I hope you'll commit to it at least for the first month or two.

It's also important to track your exercise, because doing so helps you hold yourself accountable to yourself and your goals. Tracking your exercise can also help you make changes if necessary, and keep tabs on your progress. You can use the combined food and exercise journal page in chapter 1 or the exercise-only journal page in chapter 6, or you can use a notebook, spreadsheet, calendar, or any exercise tracking app that fits your needs.

To keep things simpler, you may want to track your food and exercise in the same place. This can also help you more easily adjust your food intake to your exercise if necessary. Many of my patients find that they are hungrier after certain types of workouts, so I help them adjust their food intake to better control hunger. I will talk more about eating before and after workouts in chapter 6.

2. *Tool up for success.*

Just a few kitchen tools will make it much easier for you to stick to your eating plan: a food scale, measuring cups, and measuring spoons. These can help refresh your knowledge of portion sizes, especially when it comes to foods that are high in fats and dense carbs. (I actually keep a measuring cup in my cereal box and a tablespoon in my bag of chia seeds!) And speaking of fats, I highly recommend you invest in an olive oil sprayer, which makes it easy to use small amounts of olive oil. You can use the sprayer to squirt oil on salad, meat that's headed to the grill, or pans in which you sauté vegetables if you don't like using the sprays available at the grocery store.

If you don't already have small plates and bowls, you may want to invest in a set, because they are an easy way to keep portions under control and help you feel more satisfied, especially if you have become accustomed to large portion sizes that are actually the equivalent of two or even three or more servings. I'll tell you more about this later, but believe me, using smaller dishes really can help you eat less!

3. Write down your numbers.

Rather than relying just on your bathroom scale as a way to gauge your weight-loss success, I suggest you use a soft tape measure to keep track of your measurements. Sometimes the numbers on the scale don't move as quickly or consistently as we would like, so keeping track of monthly measurements can provide helpful motivation.

When you get started, measure your waist, hips, upper thighs, and arms, and remeasure every one or two months. If you're just starting an exercise program, you might find that your inches drop more quickly than the numbers on the scale, which means that you're losing fat and gaining muscle—a big plus when it comes to long-term weight loss.

You might also want to track your body fat. When patients come to see me, I use a specialized scale that measures their body fat. Over time, successful patients see their body fat decrease and their muscle mass increase—a very powerful motivator! If you're interested in tracking your body fat measurements at home, consider getting your own body fat scale. Just make sure to use it at the same time each day, as the measurements are very sensitive to hydration levels, which generally increase over the course of the day. You may also have the option of having your body fat measured periodically at your gym, health club, or doctor's office. If you do, you can keep track of it in your food or exercise journal, or with the Doctor on Demand app.

Finally, if you have any medical problems that may be related to excess weight, including high blood pressure, high cholesterol, or diabetes, write down those numbers, too. You will most likely see a drop in these values as you lose weight. Like many of my patients, you will certainly find that those improvements are a very powerful motivator to stay on track!

4. Seek social support.

Many studies have found that a supportive social network can improve the chances that a diet or exercise program will succeed. I urge you to try to build a network of people who support your weight-loss efforts. This can include any (or all) of the following: a health-minded friend, a doctor or nutritionist, a psychologist, a colleague at work who is also trying to slim down, an encouraging relative or spouse, a personal trainer, a neighbor looking for a walking partner, or even an online community of like-minded people with whom you feel comfortable sharing your ups and downs. The more people you have in your corner, the better your chances of success!

Now that you're all ready to get going, it's time to introduce you to Phase 1 of the Doctor on Demand Diet: the CleanStart Plan.

—ɯɯ—

Phase 1:
The CleanStart Plan

The Doctor on Demand Diet starts with a 10-day Phase 1 plan that I refer to as the CleanStart Plan. I think of this kickoff phase as a "clean start" because it promotes consistent weight loss right from the beginning, which helps reward and motivate you as you make changes to your diet and lifestyle. It also helps you "clean out" the junk food, excess sugar, excess fat, and other foods in your diet that stand between you and successful weight loss.

Strong results at the beginning of a weight-loss program pay off in the short term as well as the long term, according to many studies. For example, researchers at the University of Florida found that people who lost weight successfully at the beginning of a program lost more weight overall, kept it off longer, and were less likely to regain it compared with those who got off to a slow start.

I've seen the same thing with my patients: initial success goes a long way toward fueling their commitment to making long-term change. But it can't come at the cost of hunger—feeling famished and deprived all the time is definitely NOT a winning strategy. That's why our goal with this first phase is quite simple: *to make every calorie count in order to maximize weight loss and minimize hunger.*

I do this by choosing nutrient-dense, highly satiating foods and following some proven meal-planning strategies. CleanStart keeps calories on the low side, but because of the kinds of foods you'll be eating and the way the plan is structured, you'll feel surprisingly happy with the amount and types of food on your daily menus.

In a Hurry?

If you're anxious to see results, stay on the CleanStart Plan for longer than 10 days. It is the most ambitious of the three phases. If you'd prefer to lose weight at a slower pace, stay on CleanStart for a week and then move on to the next phase, or you can even skip it altogether.

CleanStart is designed to carry you through the first 10 days of the Doctor on Demand Diet. If you choose, you can stay on it for a second 10 days. You can also cycle back to it in the future to help kick-start weight loss, break through plateaus, or get yourself back on track. (We'll talk more about cycling in Phase 3.)

The CleanStart Daily Eating Plan

What's involved with CleanStart? I'll fill you in on it all. First, I'll start by showing you an overview of the CleanStart daily eating plan, which you'll follow for 10 days. Then, I'll explain it in detail, so that in addition to knowing *what* foods I'm recommending, you'll understand *why* I've chosen them. In the back of this book, I provide a sample menu plan that you can use as a jumping-off point for organizing your own CleanStart daily eating plans.

The CleanStart Plan Ground Rules

It's not enough just to follow a weight-loss plan. In order to succeed long-term, you do best when you understand the recommendations and philosophy used to design the plan. Knowing *why* certain food choices make more sense than others can go a long way toward helping you make the best choices at every meal. When you really understand and buy in to the ideas behind a weight-loss plan, you can embrace it and get the very most from it, both for weight loss and health.

Here are the ground rules I've used to create the CleanStart Plan. They are based on nutritional science as well as the strategies that have helped my patients meet their weight-loss goals.

The CleanStart Plan

Type of Food	Daily Servings	Sample Foods
Pure Protein	Women: 8–12 ounces per day (measured after cooking) Men: 10–14 ounces per day Note: 1 ounce = 7 grams protein	Skinless white-meat poultry Extra-lean ground white-meat poultry White fish (flounder, sole, cod, tilapia) Shellfish (shrimp, clams, scallops, lobster) Canned tuna in water Lean red meat (tenderloin, London broil, top sirloin, choice top round) Bison Extra-lean lunch meat (less than 1 gram of fat per ounce) Eggs/egg whites (1 ounce = 1 whole egg, 2 egg whites, or 1/4 cup egg substitute) Protein powder (low-sugar; 7 grams is equivalent to 1 ounce of protein)
Mixed Protein (Includes starchy protein, fatty protein, dairy protein, vegetarian protein)	Up to 5 servings per day total	**Starchy Protein** *(limit 2 servings per day; count as both a mixed protein and a dense carb)* 1/2 cup cooked beans **Fatty Protein** *(limit 1 serving per day; count as both a mixed protein and a fat)* 2 tablespoons nuts+ 1 tablespoon nut butter+ 2 tablespoons seeds+ + *Portion sizes of nuts and seeds are different when counted as protein vs. fat because they contain less protein than fat.*

Continues ▶

The CleanStart Plan (*continued*)

Type of Food	Daily Servings	Sample Foods
Mixed Protein (Includes starchy protein, fatty protein, dairy protein, vegetarian protein)	Up to 5 servings per day total	**Dairy Protein** Dairy Protein *(limit 2 servings per day)* 6 ounces plain, nonfat yogurt, preferably Greek or Iceland style 1/2 cup fat-free or low-fat cottage cheese 1 ounce low-fat hard cheese or string cheese 1/3 cup low-fat ricotta 2–3 tablespoons fresh grated Parmesan or part skim shredded mozzarella Medium-Fat Dairy Protein *(limit 1 serving per day)* 1 ounce goat cheese or mozzarella 2 tablespoons blue cheese or feta **Vegetarian Protein** Vegetarian Protein *(limit 1 serving per day unless you are a vegetarian; nuts and beans are also vegetarian protein but are listed under starchy and fatty protein)* 1 cup unsweetened soy milk 3 ounces tofu
Dense Carbs	Up to 2 servings per day	1/2 cup cooked beans *(count as both a mixed protein and a dense carb)* 1/2 cup cooked whole grains such as quinoa, brown rice, or barley* 1/2 cup cooked oats 1/2 cup starchy vegetables, such as corn, peas, or sweet potatoes **Omit if following a gluten-free diet or trial period.*

The CleanStart Plan (*continued*)

Type of Food	Daily Servings	Sample Foods
Lower-Sugar/ Higher-Fiber Fruits	Up to 2 servings per day	1 small apple/orange/pear 1/2 grapefruit 1 cup fresh or frozen berries/ sliced strawberries or 8 medium whole strawberries 1 medium peach or 1 cup frozen sliced peaches 2 apricots
Non-Starchy Vegetables	At least 5 servings per day	1/2 cup cooked or 1 cup raw fresh or frozen vegetables
Fats	Up to 3 per day	1 teaspoon olive or canola oil 1/4 avocado or 2 tablespoons guacamole 8–10 olives 2 tablespoons hummus 1 cup unsweetened almond milk or coconut milk beverage (not coconut milk, which is much higher in calories) 1 tablespoon seeds+ 1 tablespoon nuts+ + *Portion sizes of nuts and seeds are different when counted as fat vs. mixed protein because they contain more fat than protein.*
Beverages	Aim for 8 cups a day; includes water and water-based beverages such as coffee and tea	Unsweetened tea or black coffee (limit caffeinated beverages to 3 cups daily) Water (flat or sparkling, plain or fruit-infused)

CleanStart Ground Rule #1
Take Advantage of the Power of Protein

Protein really is the starting point for the Doctor on Demand Diet. I don't consider it a "high-protein diet" in the usual sense, because many of the high-protein diets out there recommend eating excessive amounts of protein and fat and fewer plant foods than I think is healthy. But I've paid a

Don't Miss Out on Mixed Protein

Some popular diets recommend cutting mixed proteins, but when it comes to weight loss and optimal health, I think this is a mistake. Here are some ways that mixed proteins come in handy:

- **Beans:** While beans are relatively high in carbohydrates, they are also loaded with hunger-busting water-soluble fiber, which helps slow the emptying of food from your stomach, control hunger, and stabilize blood sugar. Research has found that replacing calorie-dense foods with beans can help you lose weight and may also decrease your risk of diabetes and heart disease.

- **Dairy:** Studies have shown that dairy consumption, when combined with a reduced-calorie diet, leads to significantly greater fat loss (especially dangerous belly fat) and greater muscle gain, both of which are important for long-term weight loss. Plus, dairy foods are loaded with bone-building calcium and heart-healthy potassium and magnesium.

- **Nuts:** These super nutrient-dense foods are often left out of low-fat diets because of their high calorie content. Research shows that they are actually associated with lower body weight and a lower risk of heart disease, and they can increase weight loss, improve hunger control, and help people stick with their diet. I consider them an important part of the Doctor on Demand Diet.

lot of attention to the protein research that has been done during the past few years, and the studies are definitely showing that a certain amount of high-quality protein eaten throughout the day can help with weight loss.

There are three reasons for this:

1. **Protein helps keep your blood sugar stable.** When you eat carbohydrate-containing foods, your body breaks them down into simple sugar (glucose) and sends it into your bloodstream. Your pancreas, an organ located behind your stomach, produces the hormone insulin, whose job it is to usher blood sugar into your cells for energy.

Foods that break down quickly into simple sugars cause a rapid rise in your blood sugar, followed by an equally rapid fall. When blood sugar drops, low blood sugar triggers hunger and dampens your energy level and, often, your mood. This series of events can lead to cravings for sugar and carbohydrates, because sugary foods raise your blood sugar more quickly than other foods. You may have experienced this after eating a high-sugar or high-carb breakfast—a donut, pastry, or bagel with orange juice, for example. Your energy peaked initially due to the large rush of sugar you dumped into your system, but then it dropped just as rapidly, leaving you feeling hungry, low, and craving more sweets.

Our goal in all phases of the Doctor on Demand Diet is to keep blood sugar relatively stable, because that helps you control hunger and cravings. One of the best ways to do this is to include protein in your meals and snacks.

2. **Protein helps control hunger and cravings.** Calorie for calorie, protein is more filling than carbohydrates or fat. Research has shown—and I've seen it among my patients as well—that on a higher-protein diet, people eat less and feel fuller than when they eat a high-carb diet. This effect may be especially significant with a higher-protein breakfast.

3. **Protein helps you lose the right kind of weight.** Your goal is to lose fat rather than lean muscle. Various studies have shown that diets higher in protein can help you maintain muscle mass and lose more fat (especially belly fat). This is good for your metabolism, because muscle burns more calories than fat. Having less belly fat also improves your health because excess belly fat is associated with several chronic diseases.

I don't advise you to go overboard on protein, or to think that eating protein means helping yourself to large portions of fatty meats, unlimited amounts of nuts, or large portions of full-fat dairy foods. But because protein helps control hunger and keep blood sugar stable throughout the day, it can help you stick to your healthy eating plan and feel good along the way. That's why I recommend eating some form of protein with every meal and most of your snacks.

Research on Demand:
Nutrient-Dense Foods Help Curb Hunger

Poor hunger control is one of the main reasons why most weight-loss diets fail. Replacing a poor diet with a more nutritious diet not only has the power to improve your health, but it can reduce hunger pangs, according to a study published in 2010 in *Nutrition Journal*. Researchers questioned subjects who shifted from a low-nutrient diet to a high-nutrient diet. Their answers showed that when they ate a high-nutrient diet, they felt less hunger and described their hunger as being less unpleasant than when they ate a low-nutrient diet.

The bottom line: Better hunger control plus better health is a winning combination for sustained weight loss. That is precisely why the Doctor on Demand Diet is built around a nutrient-dense diet that teaches you to make every calorie count without cutting out any major food group.

Smart Protein Sources

Since protein is such a key part of the Doctor on Demand Diet, it's important for you to know what kinds of protein foods are best to include in your daily eating plan. So here's a quick explanation of what I have in mind when I talk about protein.

Protein can be found in different kinds of foods. I find it most helpful to divide protein foods into two categories: pure protein and mixed protein.

Pure proteins are foods that are made up almost entirely of protein, without too much fat and with no carbohydrates. Examples of pure proteins are lean poultry, fish, shellfish, and meat. Eggs are pure proteins because, even though yolks do contain fat (along with several important nutrients), egg whites are high in protein. In fact, they are considered to be the highest-quality dietary protein.

Mixed proteins are foods that contain a good amount of protein, but they contain more fat or carbohydrates than protein. Examples of mixed proteins are starchy proteins (beans), fatty proteins (nuts, seeds), dairy proteins (milk, cheese, yogurt, and other dairy foods), and vegetarian proteins (tofu, soy). Soy foods can be considered pure proteins if they are low in fats and carbohydrates—it depends on how they're formulated.

The Doctor on Demand Diet includes recommended amounts of pure proteins as well as mixed proteins. This helps ensure that you get the protein you need without overdoing it on calories, fat, and carbohydrates.

How Much Protein Should You Eat?

In general, I recommend that women following the CleanStart Plan eat 8 to 12 ounces of pure protein, and men 10 to 14 ounces of pure protein daily, PLUS up to five servings daily of mixed proteins. This comes out to approximately 80 to 120 grams of protein per day.

Determining exactly how many of grams of protein an individual person should eat each day is complicated business; it requires careful calculations by a nutrition expert. For our purposes, keeping to the ranges I've suggested should give you the protein you need while optimizing for weight loss, blood sugar stability, and hunger control. However, there are a few things to keep in mind:

- If you are tall (women over five feet eight inches, men over six feet) or have more than 50 pounds to lose, go to the higher end of the range.

- If you are short (women under five feet three inches, men under five feet six inches) or have less than 20 pounds to lose, stay on the lower end of the range.

- Men and women who are very physically active should stay on the higher end of the range.

- If you feel like you need more specific guidelines, consult with a dietitian or nutritionist who can make recommendations specifically for you.

Protein Choices for Vegetarians

Including protein in all meals and most snacks can be something of a challenge for vegetarians, but with some smart planning, vegetarians can follow the Doctor on Demand Diet. If you're a vegetarian, the choices you make will depend on what type of vegetarian you are.

- If you eat fish, dairy, and eggs, you will have no problem finding numerous protein choices for meals and snacks.

- If you don't eat fish, you may want to consider taking a fish oil supplement as a source of omega-3 fatty acids.

- Whether you choose to avoid dairy because of personal taste or because you are lactose-intolerant, you can make the CleanStart Plan dairy-free by replacing your two daily dairy proteins with two additional servings of pure protein or one fatty protein and one vegetarian protein if you are a vegetarian. Keep in mind, though, that many people with lactose intolerance can eat yogurt without symptoms, as yogurt contains live bacterial cultures that can help you digest lactose. Also, remember that although leafy greens can be a good source of calcium, if you don't eat dairy it's worth talking with your doctor about taking a calcium and vitamin D supplement.

- Without dairy and eggs, it can be challenging getting enough protein, especially at breakfast. Consider using a plant-based protein powder to make smoothies or add to oatmeal. Soy protein is a high-quality protein, and other plant-based protein blends can be a good choice, because the blend ensures that you get all the essential amino acids.

- If you are a total vegan and don't eat any fish, dairy, or eggs, it will be tougher to follow my recommendations because of limited lean protein options—but not impossible. Tofu is an excellent source of protein, as is protein powder. Beans and nuts are good sources of protein, but beans are high in carbohydrates, and seeds and nuts are high in fat, so you should limit oil intake if you rely on seeds and nuts for much of your protein. In place of dairy, feel free to add an additional serving or two of beans.

- If you have metabolic syndrome or elevated blood sugar, following a vegan diet will make losing weight more complicated. You may need to work with a dietitian or nutritionist to figure out how best to balance your blood sugar and get all the nutrients you need.

Research on Demand: Is Fast Best?

You may have heard that losing weight slowly is more likely to lead to long-term weight success than quick weight loss. But is this true? To test this long-held assumption, researchers compared the long-term results of three groups of obese adults: those who lost weight at a "fast" rate (at least 1.5 pounds per week), a "moderate" rate (between half a pound and 1.5 pounds per week), and a "slow" rate (under half a pound per week). The study, which was published in the *International Journal of Behavioral Medicine* in 2010, found that after six months, the people in the fast group had lost more weight (about 30 pounds) than those in the moderate group (about 20 pounds), and those in the moderate group lost more than those in the slow group (about 11 pounds). And after 18 months, those results held up: compared with the slow group, the fast group was more than five times more likely to have lost 10 percent of their weight, and the moderate group was nearly three times more likely to have lost 10 percent of their weight.

The bottom line: You have to take the approach that you feel will work best for you, and remember, your rate of weight loss depends on many factors, not just how closely you follow a diet. The CleanStart phase of the Doctor on Demand Diet is designed to help you lose weight faster initially, but that doesn't happen for everyone. If you don't lose weight quickly in the beginning, don't get discouraged. Just do your best to stick to the plan. If you feel that you are following the plan closely but losing weight very slowly, consider consulting a dietitian or nutritionist.

CleanStart Ground Rule #2
Choose Carbohydrates That Count

Carbohydrates have gotten a bad rap during the past few years. Some fad diets cut them out almost completely; others drastically limit them. I take a more reasonable approach that I believe is healthier and that I have found is much more likely to result in better long-term weight control.

The low-carb diet craze focused on cutting carbohydrates as much as possible to force your body to burn fat for fuel. Although this approach can work for quick weight loss, it often comes at the expense of considerable muscle loss, too. Plus, it's just not realistic because life without carbohydrates can be difficult to maintain and can leave you feeling tired and depressed.

The truth is, carbohydrates are not as bad as some people make them out to be. The secret is to understand the differences among the many kinds of carbohydrate foods. Some, such as most fruits, vegetables, and whole grains, are full of nutrients and are a crucial part of a healthy diet. Others are not so good, and it makes sense to cut back or eliminate them.

Our goal is to choose carbohydrate foods that are high in fiber and low in sugar (rather than those that are low in fiber and high in sugar) and to be sure to eat them with protein foods. Eating high-fiber foods helps you feel full by increasing the volume of food on your plate without adding lots of extra calories.

 ### Research on Demand: A Little Apple Goes a Long Way

This is what I call a great return on a nutritional investment. In a 2009 study in the journal *Appetite*, researchers reported that when subjects ate 125 calories worth of apple slices 15 minutes before a buffet meal, they ate about 190 calories less during the meal than those who ate nothing before the meal. Because they are processed and contain less fiber, 125 calories worth of applesauce and apple juice did not cause the same satiating effect.

The bottom line: Eating high-fiber foods such as an apple before a meal may help you eat less during the meal.

A Field Guide to Carbohydrates

Carbohydrates are found in many kinds of food. I divide them up in this way:

Dense carbs include beans, whole grains (and whole-grain products like pasta, bread, crackers, and cereal), and starchy vegetables. The dense carbs recommended on this plan are higher in fiber and lower in sugar and contain vitamins, minerals, and other nutrients. Dense carbs can keep you fuller longer and can help stabilize blood sugar, because they are broken down slowly by your body (higher-fiber foods are digested more slowly than lower-fiber foods). But dense carbs are limited throughout the Doctor on Demand Diet because they are higher in calories and carbohydrates.

Non-starchy vegetables (leafy and non-leafy) are a fantastic source of nutrients and fiber. I encourage you to eat generous amounts of non-starchy vegetables—no need even to keep count of your servings, because they are so good for you and so filling, yet add so few calories to your daily diet.

Avoid Sugar Spikes!

One way to prevent blood sugar spikes is to watch what kinds of carbs you eat. Higher-fiber/lower-sugar carbs (like oats or beans) raise blood sugar more slowly than lower-fiber/higher-sugar carbs (like a bagel or a cup of white rice), for example.

Combining carbohydrates with fat or protein can also stabilize blood sugar. For example, an apple with peanut butter (lower-sugar fruit combined with protein and fat) raises blood sugar more slowly than a cup of grapes (higher-sugar fruit without protein or fat added).

So what's the bottom line? When your blood sugar rises and falls rapidly, you are likely to feel hungry, tired, and moody. When it stays relatively stable throughout the day, you're more likely to feel physically satisfied, energetic, and emotionally positive—three very important factors when it comes to sticking with a weight-loss plan.

Fruit is included in moderate amounts in the CleanStart Plan—up to two servings per day of lower-sugar/higher-fiber fruits. Most fruits provide generous amounts of nutrients, but they also contain natural sugars and more calories than most vegetables. In my clinical experience, too much fruit can interfere with weight loss, and too much fruit sugar can get in the way of blood sugar stabilization. And I have found that many of my patients feel fuller after eating lower-sugar/higher-fiber fruits compared with higher-sugar fruits.

The fruits that I have chosen to include in the CleanStart Plan are on the list because, according to my analysis, they have the most favorable ratio of sugar to fiber—that is, they are lower in sugar and higher in fiber than other fruits. Fiber helps put the brakes on the action of sugar in your body, so in fruit, lower-sugar/higher-fiber is, in my mind, a winning combination.

In future phases of the diet, you'll have more fruit choices—but for now, it's best to stick to lower-sugar, higher-fiber choices in order to optimize for early weight loss.

Higher-sugar, lower-fiber carbohydrates are found in sugary, refined, and processed foods such as white bread, white rice, white pasta, candy, cake, fruit juice, crackers, cookies, and other foods with added sugar, corn syrup, and caloric sweeteners. You don't need these foods in your diet, so I don't include them; however, I do understand that you may occasionally want to eat them. I urge you to hold off on them for now, during the CleanStart Plan. Later, after you start losing pounds and inches, I'll show you how you can occasionally have them without jeopardizing your success.

Research on Demand: Making a Case to Cut Sugar

We Americans are eating more added sugar now than in the past, according to a study presented at the Obesity Society's 2014 annual meeting. The study showed that added sugar consumption by American adults increased by more than 30 percent, from 228 calories per day in 1977 to 300 calories in 2009–2010. If you simply cut this much sugar from your diet, you could lose over half a pound a week. Plus, excess sugar consumption is associated with an increased risk of heart disease, diabetes, fatty liver disease, and certain cancers.

The bottom line: Cut back on sugar . . . a lot! Sugar is not only found in obvious places like soft drinks and sweets, it can also be found in unexpected places like sauces, salad dressing, yogurt, and bread products, so you have to read labels to find it. And don't be fooled by healthier sounding "natural" sugars like coconut sugar, honey, organic cane sugar, agave, or brown rice syrup—for the most part, sugar is sugar, and it should be cut as much as possible during the CleanStart Plan. Don't worry, I'll let you bring a *little* sugar back during the remainder of the plan, but for now, I want to make every calorie count. Added sugar contains excess calories without any additional nutrients, so it could slow weight loss during this phase considerably.

My Challenge to You: Cut Out Dry Carbs for 10 Days

I urge all of my patients to cut back on "dry carbs" as much as possible during the CleanStart Plan. That includes bread, tortillas, crackers, pasta, and breakfast cereals (except for oatmeal). Don't worry—you can add them back, in moderation, in the next phase of the program (which is *only* 10 days away). But for now, it's incredibly beneficial for you to cut back on or, better yet, completely cut dry carbs.

Why? First of all, most of us rely far too heavily on dry carbs because they are easy and readily available. If you simply cut them out of your diet, I can almost guarantee that you will eat less and lose more without having to count calories. It's a simple step that can lead to very big results. In addition, my goal is to teach you to make every calorie count to help you control hunger better—one of the keys to staying on a diet. Dry carbs don't satisfy hunger as well as the dense carbs I recommend in this phase (beans, oats, and whole grains).

I know it seems like a bit of a sacrifice, but I asked my fans on Facebook if they would be willing to do it and the overwhelming response was yes (as long as it was just for 10 days). And it really doesn't have to be so rough: Instead of a boring bowl of cereal or a dull bagel, you can enjoy a delicious oatmeal cookie smoothie or a tasty egg white cupcake or two. And that turkey sandwich with a side of pretzels doesn't hold a candle to a super-satisfying Mexicali salad with avocado or a savory steak house salad.

If the thought of cutting out bread and pasta, even for just 10 days, makes you want to give up before you even get started, by all means include a serving or two on occasion. But to achieve the best results, challenge yourself to go "dry" for 10 days. I really do think you'll be pleasantly surprised by the results!

A Matter of Density

A concept called energy density comes into play when it comes to dry carbs. Focusing on the energy density of foods is the centerpiece of research by scientist Barbara Rolls, PhD, who created the "Volumetrics" diet plan. Foods with high energy density have higher calorie contents in relation to their total volume, and foods with lower energy density have lower calorie contents in relation to their total volume.

Energy density is based on three things: the amount of fat, fiber, and water in foods. Foods that are high in fiber and water and low in fat have lower energy density (a good thing), and foods low in water (like dry foods), low in fiber, and high in fat have a higher energy density (not as good if you are trying to feel full with fewer calories).

A good example of this is grapes and raisins. For 120 calories, you can have two cups of grapes or 1/4 cup of raisins. Although they have the same number of calories, the two cups of grapes are much more filling than the quarter cup of raisins because they contain a much higher volume of water. Another good example is strawberries: a cup of sliced strawberries has about the same number of calories (50) as a tablespoon of strawberry jam—but there's no doubt that the strawberries, which are full of both fiber and water, will fill you up way more than the jam, which contains much less water and fiber.

In my office, I use plastic models of food to visually hammer home this concept. I place a tablespoon of oil (high energy density due to high fat content, low water content, and low fiber content), one cup of cereal (medium energy density due to low fat content, low water content, and moderate fiber content), and four cups of vegetables together on my desk and explain to my patients that all three have about the same number of calories. When I ask them which of the three they think would help them feel more full, the answer is always clear: obviously having four cups of food versus a measly tablespoon of oil is going to fill you up more. It's a powerful visual lesson.

Other examples of higher-volume, lower-calorie foods include non-starchy vegetables, most fresh fruits, broth-based soups, fruit- and veggie-based smoothies, and low-fat/nonfat dairy foods.

Since the CleanStart Plan is lower in calories, I want you to have as much volume as possible to feel satisfied. Cutting dry carbs, cutting back on fat, and focusing on higher-volume, lower-calorie foods can really help with this. Almost all of the recipes I've included in this book are high volume for maximum satisfaction.

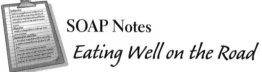

SOAP Notes
Eating Well on the Road

Monica is a busy travelling nurse in her late 50s with high blood pressure, high cholesterol, and an underactive thyroid. When she first started seeing me about four years ago, she weighed almost 300 pounds. She told me she had been a big baby and had struggled with her weight her entire life, especially during and after menopause. She swam regularly but had never done any weight training and spent a lot of time on the road and eating meals on the go. She had tried low-carb diets in the past but they always had made her feel terrible, so she quickly gave up on them. Here is a note about three months into the program, at which point she had already lost 27 pounds.

Subjective:

Patient feels great; she is not suffering and does not feel like she is on a diet. Scheduled a couple of sessions with a trainer in response to my suggestion that she exercise more intensely and add weight training; she feels the trainer really helped her push herself and do things she did not think she was capable of doing. She says eating protein as well as having a light meal in the evening are helping prevent her from getting hungry. She is seven pounds away from a weight she has not seen in 15 years. She is getting to the gym five times per week, doing cardio for 20 to 30 minutes per session and strength training twice a week.

Objective:

Patient down 10.6 pounds in the past month, and muscle mass is up slightly. Food journal analysis shows she has the same breakfast most days and rarely has a real lunch—often just has multiple snacks in the car (nuts, protein bars, string cheese, 100-calorie packs of dry snacks). Many days she does not consume adequate vegetables; twice weekly she indulges in small movie theater popcorn. Dinner is usually a salad; needs sweet treat most nights.

Assessment and Plan:

1. Exercise: Increase cardio intensity through interval training to boost calorie burning and offset drop in metabolism secondary to weight loss. Swimming is good but is not a weight-bearing activity and may not burn as many calories as other activities unless she really pushes herself.

2. Behavior: Patient seems to be in a really positive frame of mind as she nears a weight-loss milestone. I suggested she celebrate with a nonfood treat for herself, and she decided she would treat herself to a massage.

3. Inadequate vegetable intake: Make an effort to pack at least one fruit and vegetable snack in the car and limit dry snacks (such as pretzels and crackers). Explained to patient that she will likely need to cut calories slightly, as she requires fewer calories due to weight loss and decreasing the calorie density of snacks during the day will help do this without increasing hunger. Gave patient several quick and easy vegetable side dish ideas to make sure she gets at least 1½ cups of vegetables at dinner every night.

4. Snacking: Educated patient on the calories in small movie theater popcorn (400) and suggested that she bring her own if possible (air popped or 100-calorie pack of microwave popcorn).

Result:

Monica has lost a total of 112 pounds and has kept most of it off for more than two years so far.

—*Melina B. Jampolis, MD*

A Nutritional Conundrum: Should You Give Up Gluten?

Gluten is a protein found in wheat, rye, and barley. Going gluten-free is a popular dietary choice lately. Food manufacturers, restaurants, and grocery stores are highlighting their gluten-free items, and several popular diet programs are advocating that just about everyone remove all gluten from their diet.

But is this necessary?

For most of us, I don't think it is. But for 5 to 10 percent of people, cutting out gluten may be a smart choice, either because they have celiac disease or gluten sensitivity.

I do not advocate a gluten-free diet for everyone. However, I think it makes sense for some people to try taking a break from wheat- and gluten-containing foods to see how they feel without them. Also, I believe many of us rely too much on wheat products, and it's good to see how easy it actually is to reduce your reliance on them.

The CleanStart Plan is very low in gluten-containing foods simply because it cuts out dry carbs, bread, and other high-gluten foods. When you give up bread and other white/dry carbs, you automatically remove a lot of the gluten from your diet. If you'd like to try eliminating gluten for a trial period, you can do so easily while you're on the CleanStart Plan.

If you give up gluten, keep in mind that in addition to being found in bread and other obvious places, it's a hidden ingredient in countless other foods that might surprise you, including soups, soy sauce and other sauces, prepared foods, frozen dinners, and salad dressings. To learn more about what foods contain gluten, consult the Celiac Disease Foundation's website: www.celiac.org.

And remember: gluten-free doesn't necessarily equal "healthy." It doesn't mean a food is low in carbs or calories—or that it tastes good. In fact, many gluten-free breads, cakes, cookies, and other products are higher in calories, fat, and sugar and lower in fiber than similar products with gluten. When food manufacturers remove gluten, they often must add sugar, salt, fat, or gums in an attempt to give gluten-free foods the taste and texture of gluten-containing foods.

Diagnosis: Celiac Disease

A small number of the people who are bothered by gluten have celiac disease, which is an autoimmune disorder. In people with celiac disease, ingesting gluten can cause a range of unpleasant symptoms as well as long-term damage to the small intestine. This occurs because the body basically attacks the small intestine when gluten is present. Although the prevalence of celiac disease is not definitively known, it's estimated to affect at least 1 percent of Americans.

Unfortunately, many of those with celiac disease don't know they have it—in fact, according to the Celiac Disease Foundation, approximately 2.5 million Americans have undiagnosed celiac disease. For people with celiac disease, avoiding gluten is essential for preventing intestinal damage, limiting nutrient malabsorption that can lead to numerous health problems, and controlling gastrointestinal symptoms.

Millions more Americans—as many as 6 percent of the population or more—have a condition known as non-celiac gluten sensitivity (NCGS). It is a condition in which celiac-like symptoms occur in people who don't have true celiac disease.

Celiac disease and NCGS can be difficult to diagnose because they can have such a wide range of symptoms—or none at all. Among their possible signs and symptoms are:

- Abdominal pain, bloating, diarrhea, constipation
- Headaches or migraines
- Hair loss
- Anxiety, irritability, depression, chronic fatigue
- Bone or joint pain; bone loss or osteoporosis
- Attention problems or a lack of mental clarity often referred to as "foggy mind"

- Unexplained iron-deficiency anemia or other nutrient deficiencies
- An itchy skin rash called dermatitis herpetiformis

If you have any of these symptoms—or if you have other autoimmune diseases (like Hashimoto's disease, a common cause of low thyroid function; rheumatoid arthritis; lupus; or multiple sclerosis) that are associated with an increased risk of celiac disease—it's a good idea to ask your doctor about having a celiac disease blood test. It is essential that you do not cut gluten prior to your blood test, as eliminating gluten can make test results less reliable. If you have an autoimmune disease and you test negative, you may want to try cutting gluten out for 10 days to see how you feel.

Vegetables and Fruit: Your Best Bets

As I said, carbohydrates have gotten a bad rap lately from some diet "experts." What they sometimes forget to mention is that some of the most nutritious foods of all—vegetables and fruits—contain carbohydrates. That doesn't mean we should avoid them—just the opposite, in fact. Vegetables and fruit are an important part of a healthy diet, and they can play a crucial role in weight loss.

Let's start with vegetables. Although there is no such thing as an unhealthy vegetable, some vegetables are better choices than others because they offer a rich array of nutrients and fiber with a relatively small number of calories. Here's how we keep track of vegetables in the Doctor on Demand Diet:

Non-starchy vegetables are so nutritious and so low in calories that you *should* eat at least five servings a day, and you *can* eat as many as you like without counting servings or portion sizes.

Starchy vegetables are also good sources of nutrients, but they contain more carbohydrates. This puts them in the category of dense carbs, which should be limited to up to two daily.

Be sure to check out the recipe section of this book, where you'll find ideas for incorporating all kinds of vegetables into soups, smoothies, salads, and other delicious menu items.

Non-starchy vegetables in the CleanStart Plan include:

- Artichokes
- Artichoke hearts
- Asparagus
- Bean sprouts
- Broccoli
- Brussels sprouts
- Cabbage
- Carrots
- Cauliflower
- Celery
- Cucumber
- Eggplant
- Green beans
- Green onions
- Green peppers
- Kale
- Leeks
- Mushrooms
- Mustard greens
- Okra
- Onions
- Pea pods
- Peppers
- Pure tomato sauce (not spaghetti sauce or marinara sauce, which may contain added fats and sugars)
- Radishes
- Red peppers
- Salad greens (endive, escarole, radicchio, lettuce, romaine)
- Spinach
- Swiss chard
- Tomatoes
- Water chestnuts
- Watercress
- Zucchini

Starchy vegetables in the CleanStart Plan include:

- Beets
- Butternut squash
- Corn
- Peas
- Sweet potato
- Turnips

Note: White potatoes are a starchy vegetable, but they are not included in the CleanStart Plan. You can include them in your diet in small quantities during later phases of the Doctor on Demand Diet.

Clinical Pearl: *Make a Plan*

Take some time to sit down every Sunday and map out your week. Go grocery shopping, plan your meals (at home and out of the house), schedule workouts in your calendar, and cook or bake meals that you can heat and eat easily on hectic weeknights. The more you plan, the greater your odds of success. ◇

The Smartest Way to Eat Fruit

Fruit is a good source of fiber, it's relatively low in calories, and it's full of vitamins, minerals, and phytonutrients. That doesn't mean you can eat unlimited amounts of it, however. Fruits that are higher in naturally occurring fruit sugar and lower in fiber can impact blood sugar and may not be as satisfying. While fruits are lower in calories than most foods, they still have calories, which can add up and may slow weight loss.

In addition to limiting your fruit intake to two servings daily, follow these steps to make sure you aren't getting too many calories from fruit:

Skip the fruit juice. Fruit juice does not contain fiber, which is important for fullness, keeping blood sugar more stable, and weight loss. Juice is also a concentrated form of calories that can be quickly consumed. Think about the amount of time that it takes you to eat an orange versus the amount of time it takes to drink a four-ounce glass of juice.

The dirty little secret about fruit juice—even 100 percent pure fruit juice—is that it contains enormous amounts of sugar and calories. For example, 100 percent pure orange juice has more calories than an equal amount of Coke, Pepsi, or other sugary soda. Sure, the orange juice has vitamin C, but if you're eating a healthy diet you're getting plenty of vitamin C from other sources, such as whole fruits and vegetables.

If you really love pure fruit juice, you can include it in small quantities in future phases of the Doctor on Demand Diet. But for now, avoid it. In my mind, juice has no place in a weight-loss program because it provides so little return on your caloric investment.

Stay away from dried fruit. Unlike juice, dried fruit contains fiber, but it does not contain water, so dried fruit is a much more concentrated source

On average, Americans consume only half the recommended daily intake of fiber (21–25 grams for women, 30–38 grams for men). But the fact is, it's super easy for everyone to reach daily fiber goals on the Doctor on Demand Diet. Here's an example of how it adds up:

Breakfast: Smoothie with 1 cup berries (3 grams) and 1 tablespoon chia seeds (5 grams) + protein powder for breakfast = 8 grams fiber

Lunch: Salad with 2 cups romaine (2 grams) + 1 cup veggies (4 grams) + 1/2 cup kidney beans (8 grams) + chicken = 14 grams

Dinner: Fish + 2 cups broccoli (5 grams) + 1/2 cup quinoa (2.5 grams) + 1/2 cup mushrooms (2.5 grams) = 10 grams

Snack: Apple (3 grams) + 2 tablespoons nuts (2 grams) = 5 grams

Total: 37 grams of fiber

of calories and sugar that can add up fast. Dried fruit falls into the same category as the dry carbs that I mentioned above—it has a higher energy density so you just don't get a lot of bang for your buck in terms of volume and hunger control. I'm always astounded by the number of calories in dried fruit: half a cup of raisins, for example, contains 240 calories—as much as a McDonald's hamburger and more than a bag of chocolate candies. Fresh fruit is also far more satisfying: for the same number of calories, you can eat two cups of grapes or a quarter cup of raisins. So stick with the whole fruit, save calories, *and* feel fuller!

CleanStart Ground Rule #3
Respect the Power of Fat

Like carbohydrates, fats have gotten a bad reputation over the past few decades. In the 1980s and early 1990s, fat was seen as a nutrition villain that should, as much as possible, be eliminated from the diet. As a result, many big food companies cut the fat in their cookies, crackers, ice cream, and frozen dinners and marketed them as healthier choices than full-fat foods. They had to replace the fat with something, and often that something was some form of highly processed sweetener, refined grains, or even salt to improve the taste.

Clinical Pearl: *Know Your Spoons*

When it comes to fats, measuring precisely really makes a difference. If you don't have a good set of measuring spoons, I recommend you get some. Using your kitchen flatware to measure fats can get you into trouble, because the teaspoons and tablespoons in your drawer may deliver larger amounts of fat than well-calibrated measuring spoons. And while you're at it, keep this in mind:

- 1 tablespoon = 3 teaspoons
- 2 tablespoons = 1/8 cup
- 4 tablespoons = 1/4 cup

Since then, we've learned that healthy fats play an important role in good health, and cutting out all fats from your diet isn't a smart strategy. For example, eating fat helps your body absorb certain vitamins. And fat actually surrounds almost every cell in your body, so it plays an essential role in optimal health.

In fact, while your body can produce some of the fat that you need from protein and carbs, there are a group of fats known as essential fatty acids that you can only get through the food you eat. They are critical for healthy brain function and vision and if you don't get enough you may develop a rash, increased risk of infection, or poor wound healing. And super-healthy essential fats such as omega-3 fatty acids can lower risk of heart attack and stroke, reduce inflammation, and may reduce your chances of developing certain kinds of cancer.

That's why the Doctor on Demand Diet includes a range of healthy fats from foods such as healthy oils (olive, canola), nuts, seeds, olives, fatty fish, and avocados.

Researchers are also investigating the positive role healthy fats may play in combatting depression, Alzheimer's disease, rheumatoid arthritis, and other health conditions. If you cut way back on dietary fat, you run the risk of vitamin deficiencies, a drop in "good" cholesterol levels, and dry skin, as well as an elevated risk of heart disease in some people. What's more, research shows that replacing some carbs with healthy fats can help improve insulin resistance—I'll tell you more about that in the next phase.

Despite that good news about fat, it's still important not to eat too much of it. All fats—even the healthiest of fats—are high in calories (more than double the calories of protein or carbs), so it's critical to watch your serving sizes closely, since calories from fats add up fast. I've seen so many patients gain weight or hit endless plateaus because they didn't bother measuring high-fat foods such as olive oil or nuts when preparing meals and snacks. For now, know that it's a good idea to eat healthy fats, but it's also important to stick to your limits, or you may find yourself not losing weight.

CleanStart Ground Rule #4
Eat Often to Lose More

I recommend that you eat every three to four hours. This makes sense for many reasons:

Frequent eating helps keep blood sugar stable. When you eat several smaller meals throughout the day rather than two or three large meals, your blood sugar level remains more stable, because you are not taking in large quantities of food followed by long periods without food. Stabilizing blood sugar keeps your energy more constant throughout the day and minimizes sugar cravings. Eating more frequently seems to be particularly important for women, who often report feeling less hungry and less moody when they eat throughout the day.

Frequent eating helps maintain muscle mass and metabolism. When we cut back on calories, our bodies sometimes react by slowing down our metabolism and using lean muscle mass for fuel. However, when people following a lower-calorie diet eat frequently—five or six times a day rather than two or three—they experience less of a drop in metabolism and muscle mass, especially if they are consuming protein throughout the day. The main reason for this is likely due to the fact that eating actually boosts metabolism slightly because the digestion of food burns calories. Plus, the digestion of protein boosts metabolism the most. (Another great reason to eat protein throughout the day!) Maintaining muscle mass and optimizing your metabolism are important both for weight loss and overall health.

Frequent eating helps prevent hunger. Spacing meals and snacks just a few hours apart allows you to feel less hungry than if you eat infrequently. This is important because it is much harder to make smart choices at

Eat Frequently—But Only When You're Hungry

I recommend eating three meals and two snacks (one mini and one full) per day. You can personalize your own meal/snack schedule, planning snacks for the times of day that you feel most hungry—in the morning, midafternoon, or evening.

There's one caveat here: don't eat if you are not hungry. This is a common mistake that I see in my patients. Some people may not get as hungry during certain times of the day or after certain meals, so never force yourself to eat—but don't let yourself get too hungry, either.

Counting calories isn't really part of my program. If you go by the serving sizes I recommend, there's no reason to tabulate calorie counts. However, I know some people like to keep track of numbers, so for those of you keeping score, here's the approximate calorie breakdown of the CleanStart Plan:

- Breakfast, about 200–300 calories
- Lunch, about 250–350 calories
- Dinner, about 300–400 calories
- Mini snack, about 100 calories
- Full snack, about 150–200 calories

meals and snacks when you are famished, as anyone who has scarfed down an entire restaurant bread basket in seconds flat can attest. You simply feel more in control when you're not fighting off huge hunger pangs.

CleanStart Ground Rule #5
Make Water Your Go-To Beverage

Drinking water helps fill you up, and studies show that it can help with weight loss, so I recommend having eight calorie-free beverages each day. These include:

- Sparkling or flat water. Add flavor by infusing it with fresh fruit (citrus slices or berries are terrific for this), herbs (such as mint), or vegetables (cucumber water is delicious).

Clinical Pearl: *The Science of Satiety*

The science behind satiety (fullness) and hunger control is complicated and involves ongoing cross talk between your gut and your brain. Numerous hormones are involved in satiety, including leptin, ghrelin, insulin, cortisol, NPY, GLP-1, CCK, and PYY, to name a few. Each person varies in his or her response to these hormones, so there is no one-size-fits-all approach to satiety strategies. However, feeling full starts with eating regular, balanced, minimally processed meals built around protein and fiber-rich whole foods. Throughout the Doctor on Demand Diet, I will give you lots of practical diet, exercise, and behavior tips that will help you manage hormones that control hunger. ◆

- Unsweetened coffee or tea. If you like coffee or tea with milk, add a touch of low-fat or fat-free milk or nondairy milk substitute with no sugar added. If, like me, you must have a sweetener, consider stevia, which is my top choice.

- Skip all sugar-sweetened beverages, including flavored waters, sports drinks, sweetened tea, and soda. These are loaded with empty calories and simply don't belong on any weight-loss plan.

- As for artificially sweetened beverages such as diet soda, I recommend avoiding them during the CleanStart Plan. If you really can't live without them, cut back as much as possible.

- I don't recommend drinking milk (or nondairy milk substitute) as a beverage during this phase. (A splash in your coffee is okay, but sorry, no lattes—they're not as filling as other foods with similar calorie counts.) Even though milk contains nutrients, liquid calories are not as satisfying as pureed or solid calories, and during this first phase of the plan I want every calorie to satisfy you as much as possible. *Note: You can have milk or a milk substitute in your morning smoothie, but just don't drink it as a beverage on its own.*

❧ Alcohol is not included in the CleanStart Plan. I leave it out because it contributes excess calories to your diet, and during this first 10 days I think it's more important to see some exciting results than to indulge in an occasional glass of wine, bottle of beer, or cocktail. If you'd rather not eliminate alcohol for this phase, just try to cut back as much as possible, and be aware that your weight loss may be slightly slower because of it.

CleanStart Ground Rule #6:
Get Out and Walk

Exercise is crucial for weight loss and good overall health. But for the 10 days that you follow the CleanStart Plan, we're going to focus primarily on your diet. We'll talk more about exercise later in the book.

Here's why: As you begin the CleanStart Plan, it doesn't make sense to launch an ambitious exercise program at the exact same time. Making lots of changes all at once can be difficult, and combining a brand-new high-intensity exercise program with a brand-new, lower-calorie eating plan can leave you feeling hungry, worn out, and unmotivated. This is a recipe for weight-loss failure.

While you're on the CleanStart Plan, I suggest you stick with whatever exercise you're currently doing. (If you are already doing high-intensity exercise, such as spinning, swimming, or running for longer than 30 minutes, you may want to add one extra fruit or dense carb to your daily meal plan if you're getting too hungry on the CleanStart Plan.)

If you're not currently doing any exercise at all, I recommend walking. A good goal is 30 minutes a day of moderate walking, but this can be too much for people who are sedentary or obese. Even 10 minutes of daily walking or a couple of short walks each day can move you in the right direction.

Counting steps is a great way to increase activity. Wearing a step counter or fitness tracking device allows you to challenge yourself every day and get "credit" for every step you take. You can go as high-tech as you want—many fitness tracking devices have apps that allow you to track your steps on your phone or computer, compete with friends, and keep track of steps over time. For some of my patients, using a step counter has made a huge difference. I have to admit that I'm kind of obsessed with my fitness tracker and I often find myself looking for any opportunity I can to walk more, especially on days where my step count is low.

If you don't currently exercise, or if you have any health problems or medical conditions, be sure to talk with your health-care provider before starting an exercise program.

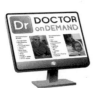

Research on Demand:
Walking Burns Fat, Lowers Blood Sugar

You don't have to run marathons to see health benefits from exercise. According to research such as a 2014 study published in the *Journal of Exercise Nutrition and Biochemistry*, moderate amounts of walking deliver impressive results. In the study, one group of obese women walked at a brisk pace 50 to 70 minutes a day, three days a week. The other maintained their previous sedentary lifestyle. After 12 weeks, researchers found that the walking group had significantly less over-all body fat and belly fat than the sedentary group. Walkers also had lower levels of blood sugar, insulin resistance, and inflammation compared to the non-active group.

The bottom line: Your whole body can benefit when you embark on a walking program. If you are new to exercise, start with just 10 minutes a day of easy walking; as you become more fit, you can walk faster, farther, and more frequently.

Planning Your CleanStart Meals

Now that you understand the gist of the CleanStart Plan, let's look at how to use it to create a daily meal plan. The CleanStart meal plans give you *both* structure and flexibility. Their structure comes from the CleanStart daily eating plan, which recommends how many (and which kinds) of pro-teins, fats, and carbohydrates to eat each day. Their flexibility comes from the freedom you have to construct meals in ways that best suit your prefer-ences, favorite food choices, and hungry times.

For best results, I recommend three meals, one mini snack, and one full snack per day. This is the structure that seems to work best for most of my patients, because it allows them to eat something every few hours.

The CleanStart Suggested Daily Meal Plan

Breakfast:
- 1 dairy protein (or 2–3 pure proteins)
- 1 fruit or dense carb
- 1 fat

Lunch:
- 3–4 proteins (pure protein or combination of pure and mixed protein)
- 2–3 vegetables
- 1 dense carb (optional)
- 1 fat

Dinner:
- 3–5 proteins (pure protein or combination of pure and mixed protein)
- 2–3 vegetables
- 1 dense carb (optional)
- 1 fat

Full Size Snack:
- 1 dairy protein (or 1–2 pure proteins)
- PLUS 1 fruit or vegetable

Mini Snack/Dessert:
- 1 dairy protein (or 1–2 pure proteins)
- OR 1 fruit
- OR 1/2 to 1 fruit + 1/2 dairy protein

Or make it your way with any of these modifications:
- Skip the fat at breakfast and have an extra fat at lunch or dinner.
- Like dense carbs with every meal? Split one serving of dense carbs into two and have half at breakfast and half at lunch.
- Need an extra snack? Cut one pure protein from dinner and combine with vegetables for a third snack.
- Don't do dairy? Have one to two pure proteins for snacks instead.
- Like something sweet at lunch? Have fruit with lunch instead of a dense carb.
- Add a non-starchy vegetable to any meal or snack to make it more satisfying.

For a 10-Day CleanStart Sample Menu, see the Menu section at the back of this book.

(You may also split your full snack into two smaller snacks, for three meals and three mini snacks per day.) You may eat your snacks midmorning, midafternoon, or in the evening, depending on when you are hungriest. Frequent eating helps keep hunger at bay, contributes to stable blood sugar, and minimizes food cravings.

Our goal with the CleanStart Plan is to distribute your foods fairly evenly throughout the day, designing a daily meal plan that includes the recommended amounts of the various choices on your CleanStart foods list.

In my experience, some people like designing their own daily meal plans, and some like to have it all figured out for them. Either way is fine, as long as you stick to the recommendations on number of daily servings, serving sizes, and so on. If you like using a step-by-step menu, refer to the one at the back of this book. Feel free to mix and match the meals and snacks provided there to create your own daily menu, but just be sure to stick to your daily limits.

The CleanStart phase is lower in both fat and dense carbohydrates than other phases of the Doctor on Demand Diet. To keep things as simple as possible, most meals contain one fat serving, and two of the three meals can contain one dense carb serving. No fat or dense carbs are included in snacks. They will be added in during the next phase.

You can use the following guide to plan CleanStart meals. This is the most common way that Doctor on Demand users choose to allocate their proteins, fat, and carbs. You can also use one of the modification options below, or design your own daily eating schedule. Just remember to include protein with all meals and most/all snacks, and to pay especially careful attention to how much fat and how many dense carbs you eat each day.

Keeping a Food and Exercise Journal

Remember I suggested that you keep a daily food and exercise journal in which you track your food intake and exercise each day? If you haven't already started doing this, now's the time to get going. Here's a handy template you can copy and use every day.

Doctor on Demand Food and Exercise Journal Page

Date: ____/____/____   Mon   Tues   Wed   Thu   Fri   Sat   Sun

Breakfast: Time _____

_____

_____

_____

Morning Snack: Time _____

_____

_____

_____

Lunch: Time _____

_____

_____

_____

Afternoon Snack: Time _____

_____

_____

Dinner: Time _____

_____

_____

_____

Evening Snack: Time _____

_____

_____

DAILY TOTALS:

Dense Carbs _____ Pure Protein _____

Dairy Protein _____ Fatty Protein _____ Starchy Protein _____

Vegetarian Protein _____ Fat _____ Fruit _____

Vegetables _____ Water: _____

(Do not forget to check off fatty protein and starchy protein in both sections)

Doctor on Demand Food and
Exercise Journal Page (*continued*)

Exercise:

Cardio: (type, duration) _____

_____

_____

_____

_____

_____

Strength Training: (sets, reps, body parts worked)

_____

_____

_____

_____

_____

Notes: _____

_____

_____

_____

_____

_____

_____

_____

_____

_____

_____

_____

_____

_____

_____

Coming Up Next: Customize Your Carbs

Once you complete Phase 1 by spending 10 days (or however long you choose) on the CleanStart Plan, you'll be ready to move on to Phase 2 of the Doctor on Demand Diet—the Customize Your Carbs Plan. In this phase, I'll explain how to customize your diet plan based on how your body responds to carbohydrates.

CHAPTER 2

—ɱ—

Phase 2:
The Customize Your Carbs Plan

Now that you have completed the CleanStart Plan, Phase 1 of the Doctor on Demand Diet, you should be seeing some encouraging results. You've likely lost anywhere from two to five pounds, and you've made great progress in "cleaning up" your diet by getting back in touch with proper portion sizes, cutting out unhealthy foods and beverages, and adding in a bounty of foods that are good for your health and your weight. You're on the right track, and now you're ready to move on to Phase 2 of the Doctor on Demand Diet.

(Note: If you enjoyed the CleanStart Plan and would like to continue it for an additional 10 days, feel free to do so. However, if you'd like to introduce slightly more flexibility to your meal plan and customize your diet to fit your health and lifestyle, continue on to Phase 2.)

The focus of this second phase is *customization.* I've found that the best way to start customizing an eating plan for success is to focus on carbohydrates—which is why Phase 2 is called the Customize Your Carbs Plan. In this part of the program, we will use information about your health to determine your best strategy for including carbohydrates and fat in your diet.

Why the emphasis on carbohydrates and fat? Because they wield a lot of power. By fine-tuning your carbohydrate and fat intake, you can take even more control of your hunger, your blood sugar, your metabolism, and ultimately, your weight-loss success.

Overall, the Customize Your Carbs Plan is slightly higher in calories and has a little more variety than the CleanStart Plan. During this second phase, you can reintroduce bread and dry carbs (in moderation), consume a greater variety of fruit, and choose from a more expanded list of protein foods that includes some higher-fat options on occasion.

I recommend following the Customize Your Carbs Plan for 10 days (or longer). After that, we'll move on to Phase 3 of the Doctor on Demand Diet. In that phase, the Cycle for Success Plan, I'll work with you to make your eating plan even more flexible and livable by showing you how to use a strategy I refer to as Diet-Cycling. More about this later—for now, let's focus on the Customize Your Carbs phase.

Customize Your Carbs: Two Tracks for Customized Success

The Customize Your Carbs Plan has two tracks. One is for people who are insulin-responsive—their bodies produce and use insulin in a normal way. The second is for people who are insulin-resistant—their bodies are resistant to the action of insulin.

Like many people, you may not have a clue how your body uses insulin. That's OK—I've included a handy quiz that will help you determine whether you are *likely* to be insulin-resistant (only a doctor can make a definitive diagnosis) and help you decide which track of the Customize Your Carbs Plan is best for you.

Like the CleanStart Plan, the Customize Your Carbs Plan is designed to be a moderately high-protein, high-fiber, low-glycemic, high-volume eating plan. The Insulin-Responsive track (for people with normal insulin response) includes slightly less fat and more carbohydrates than the Insulin-Resistant track, which is slightly higher in fat and lower in carbohydrates.

Customize Your Carbs also makes space for the reintroduction of bread (provided you don't have celiac disease or gluten intolerance/sensitivity) and other dry carbs, although I do recommend that you consume them in limited amounts because they tend to be lower-volume/higher-calorie foods. If you are insulin-resistant, I suggest you limit bread intake to one serving per day. You can also reintroduce your beloved caffe latte as long as you keep it small, have it prepared with nonfat or low-fat milk, count it as part of a meal or snack, and skip the sugary syrups.

SOAP Notes

Facing the Economic Challenges of Healthy Eating

Carmen is a 32-year-old diabetic with an obese 4-year-old daughter. I began seeing Carmen a few years ago as part of a volunteer community outreach program that I started. She weighed 330 pounds, had very poorly controlled diabetes, could not afford all of her diabetes medications, worked full time, and relied mainly on food stamps to feed her family. Here is a note from one of my early consultations with her.

Subjective:

Patient is struggling to eat healthy dinners due to lack of time and money. She has cut out fruit juice and began getting off the bus to and from work one stop early to increase exercise, and even managed to walk home from work one day (30 minutes).

Objective:

Weight unchanged from two weeks ago. Food journal limited, but when asked to recall meals in previous 24 hours she described cream of wheat and egg for breakfast, a wrap for lunch, a ground-beef casserole for dinner, and limited vegetable intake.

Assessment and Plan:

1. Breakfast: Suggested switch to oatmeal for breakfast instead of cream of wheat to add fiber. Suggested that patient make a big pot of slow-cooked oats to heat and eat throughout the week.

2. Dinner: Advised patient to look for lower-fat meats on sale at the store and buy in bulk and freeze, because regular ground beef can be very high in fat and calories. Suggested that patient cut back on cheese in casserole and try to add in spices and vegetables such as onions and garlic to boost flavor instead.

3. Vegetable intake: Boost with frozen (no sauce added) and even canned vegetables on sale. While romaine lettuce is a better choice for salads, iceberg lettuce is OK if that's all that is available or that she can afford— just watch the dressing serving size. Encouraged patient to look for measuring spoons and cups at a dollar store so she can pay closer attention to portions of dense carbs such as pasta, rice, cereal, oats, oils, and fats.

4. Encouraged patient to keep increasing lifestyle exercise such as getting off the bus two stops early when possible and walking errands with her daughter on weekends when she has more time.

Result:

Over the course of two years, Carmen lost more than 90 pounds. Her diabetes control improved and she was able to reduce her insulin dose significantly. She has moved away, but keeps in touch and is continuing to lose slowly on her own.

—*Melina B. Jampolis, MD*

Insulin: A Major Influence on Weight and Health

In Phase 2 of the Doctor on Demand Diet, we talk a lot about insulin. Why? Because how your body uses insulin can have a huge impact on your weight and your health. Determining whether you have insulin resistance is one of the most important aspects of finding the weight-loss strategy that will be the most effective for you.

Before we move on, let's make sure you understand the concept of insulin resistance and its relation to blood sugar, overall health, and weight loss. It's a bit confusing, but I'll do my best to explain it in the clearest way possible.

As we discussed earlier in the book, insulin is a hormone produced by the pancreas, an organ located in your abdomen near your liver. Insulin plays an important role in your body's metabolism, which is the collective name for all of the biological processes your body uses to convert food into fuel, and to use that fuel for energy.

When you eat food, your body breaks down the food's carbohydrates into glucose, a form of simple sugar that serves as fuel for your cells. As glucose is produced, it enters your bloodstream. If a doctor takes a sample of your blood shortly after you eat a meal containing carbohydrates, the test would show that your blood glucose (or blood sugar) level is elevated.

As glucose enters your bloodstream, insulin release is triggered in your pancreas and insulin is pumped into your blood. Insulin's job is to usher the glucose in the blood to your muscle, liver, and fat cells. As cells take glucose from your blood, levels of glucose and insulin in your blood go back down to normal levels.

That's how it's *supposed* to happen—but in some people, this process doesn't go quite as smoothly as it should, and their bodies start responding less well to insulin. In the bodies of people with insulin resistance, insulin doesn't work as effectively as it's supposed to—kind of like a key not working correctly to unlock a door. When insulin can't do its job of bringing glucose to cells, glucose builds up in the blood. (People with normal insulin response are described as being insulin-responsive.) In addition, your cells are not receiving the glucose that they need to burn for energy, which can make you feel tired and hungry.

When Insulin Doesn't Work

In people who have insulin resistance, the pancreas keeps producing more and more insulin in an effort to move glucose out of the blood and bring blood sugar levels down. This can be a major problem if you are trying to lose weight because insulin has another job: to promote fat storage and prevent fat breakdown. If you are insulin-resistant and regularly consume foods that increase blood sugar and insulin levels (the wrong carbohydrates or too many carbohydrates), it can be very difficult for you to lose fat.

Get Moving to Stabilize Blood Sugar

Being sedentary raises the risk of elevated blood sugar for several reasons: you have less muscle to process glucose, and inactive muscles are less responsive to insulin and use up *less* glucose, causing glucose to build up in the blood. When you exercise, several things happen that are good for blood sugar and insulin levels:

- Exercise builds muscle, so having more muscle cells means that you use more glucose, which can help maintain healthy blood sugar levels.
- Active muscles use more blood glucose for fuel than inactive muscles.
- With regular exercise, your muscles become more sensitive to the action of insulin, making your body less insulin-resistant even if you don't lose weight!

Clinical Pearl: *Turn Down the Burn*

Inflammation is strongly associated with visceral obesity (belly fat) and insulin resistance. The type of inflammation I'm talking about is not the inflammation that occurs when you skin your knee and your body produces inflammatory cells that rush to the site to help you heal. That kind of inflammation is good for you, because it heals wounds. Worrisome inflammation is chronic (ongoing) and low-grade (simmering) and can actually damage healthy cells and cause lots of problems in your body.

How can you fight this kind of unhealthy inflammation? By cutting back on proinflammatory foods, including refined carbohydrates, sugar, and saturated fat, and by eating a diet that is rich in anti-inflammatory omega-3 fatty acids as well as colorful fruits and vegetables, beans, nuts, and spices. Anti-inflammatory foods contain powerful substances that help fight inflammation.

Insulin resistance is also associated with leptin resistance. Leptin is a hormone produced by fat that acts in the brain to suppress appetite and increase metabolism. Resistance to leptin can make weight loss even more challenging.

Over time in people with insulin resistance, the pancreas can lose its ability to produce enough insulin, and blood glucose levels remain high (commonly known as having high blood sugar). As a result, type 2 diabetes can develop. Having chronically high blood glucose can damage blood vessels, organs, and nerves. Insulin resistance can also raise the risk of developing diseases of the heart, liver, kidneys, brain, and even certain types of cancer.

Unfortunately, many people don't know they have insulin resistance. They don't discover it until their doctors diagnose diabetes (an often permanent condition in which average blood glucose levels are too high) or prediabetes (a potentially reversible condition in which average blood glucose levels are higher than normal, but not high enough to be considered diabetes).

Doctors and scientists don't know exactly what causes insulin resistance. However, there do seem to be strong connections between insulin

Clinical Pearl: Shape Up Your Gut

New and evolving research shows that the standard American diet, which is high in sugar and saturated fat and low in fiber, causes changes in the number and type of bacteria in your gut. Changes can happen as quickly as 24 hours after eating a high-fat meal and can lead to inflammation and alterations in your metabolism that can actually cause weight gain and contribute to insulin resistance. To get your gut back in shape, cut back on sugar and saturated fat and boost your intake of fermented foods like yogurt, kefir, tempeh, and miso soup that contain beneficial bacteria known as probiotics. It's also critical to boost your intake of fruits and vegetables because they are loaded with prebiotic fiber and polyphenols, which help support the healthy bacteria in your gut. To learn more about this fascinating new area of nutrition, check out *The Gut Balance Revolution* by my colleague Gerard E. Mullin, MD. ◈

resistance and being overweight, having excess belly fat, and being physically inactive.

Belly fat produces hormones and inflammatory cells (called cytokines) that contribute to insulin resistance. Having excess belly fat increases inflammation in the body, which plays a key role in insulin resistance; burning off belly fat through changes in diet and exercise can reduce inflammation and insulin resistance and lower the risk of type 2 diabetes.

In addition, insulin resistance is more common in people who smoke, have sleep apnea, work night shifts, take certain medications such as steroids, and come from high-risk ethnic groups.

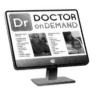 ## Research on Demand: Yogurt May Reduce Diabetes Risk

Not only is yogurt packed with protein, but it may help prevent type 2 diabetes, according to a 2014 study published in the journal *Diabetologia*. The study found that compared with people who did not eat yogurt, people who ate about 20 ounces of yogurt a week had a 28 percent lower risk of developing type 2 diabetes. Researchers believe yogurt's high levels of vitamin D, calcium, and magnesium, as well as its beneficial probiotic bacteria, offer protection against diabetes.

The bottom line: There are many reasons to include low-fat or fat-free yogurt in your diet, including its potential to lower diabetes risk. It's an important component of the Doctor on Demand Diet. Just make sure to watch the sugar content—some yogurts have as much sugar as a candy bar. If you don't love the tart taste of some yogurt, mix in crushed fresh berries, a little no-calorie sweetener, or a teaspoon of honey. Give it some time and you may come to love it.

Prediabetes: A Reversible Risk

Prediabetes is exactly what it sounds like: a condition that develops before diabetes. It occurs in people whose blood sugar levels are higher than they should be, but not high enough to be considered diabetes. Approximately 86 million American adults have prediabetes; they are at an increased risk of developing type 2 diabetes, heart disease, and strokes.

The good news about prediabetes is that it is often reversible. Studies have shown that losing just 5 to 10 percent of your body weight can prevent or delay the onset of diabetes. For someone who weighs 200 pounds, that's a weight loss of 10 to 20 pounds—which is really not that much weight.

Scientists have found that people with prediabetes are at high risk for developing type 2 diabetes within about 10 years unless they make important changes to their diet, weight, and exercise levels.

Unfortunately, prediabetes has no symptoms. The only way to know if you have it is to have your blood glucose levels tested by a health-care provider. According to the National Diabetes Information Clearinghouse, you should be tested for prediabetes if, *in addition to being overweight*, you:

- Are physically inactive
- Have a parent or sibling with diabetes
- Have high blood pressure or high cholesterol
- Have low HDL ("good") cholesterol
- Had gestational diabetes (pregnancy diabetes) or a baby weighing more than nine pounds

- Are African American, Alaska Native, American Indian, Asian American, Hispanic/Latino, or Pacific Islander American

- Have polycystic ovary syndrome (PCOS)

- Have a dark, velvety rash around your neck or armpits

- Have blood vessel problems affecting your brain, heart, or lungs

If you're not sure whether you should have your blood sugar checked, I recommend that you do so, especially if you're overweight, over age 45, or haven't had it tested in the past few years. If you have prediabetes or, even more importantly, diabetes, you should know about it.

Diabetes is a serious health condition that can lead to kidney failure, blindness, and amputations, and it significantly increases your risk of heart disease. It can be controlled with diet, exercise, and medication. But the first step is diagnosis, and unfortunately, many people who have it don't know it. In the United States, over 29 million people (9.3 percent of the population) have diabetes—but of those, approximately 8.1 million (28 percent) have not been diagnosed. See your doctor to arrange for a diabetes blood test.

 Clinical Pearl: *Go for the Green*

Leafy greens are super low in calories and loaded with fiber, vitamins and minerals, and powerful phytonutrients called carotenoids. Just a little more than one serving per day can decrease your risk of diabetes by 14 percent, and regular consumption may also lower your risk of heart disease and possibly certain types of cancer. They also can help promote bone, skin, and eye health. Add greens into soups, salads, scrambled eggs, smoothies, and stir-fries. For details, see the Recipe section of this book. ◇

Steps to Improve Insulin Resistance

If you are insulin-resistant, there are many steps you can take to improve your condition. The following are some of the simple things you can do—or avoid doing—to have an impact on your insulin function.

Factors That Contribute to Insulin Resistance

- Eating too much saturated fat
- Consuming too many high-sugar foods, especially sugar-sweetened beverages
- Having poor sleep habits
- Eating a low-fiber diet
- Smoking
- Taking certain medications, including steroids, some antidepressants, mood stabilizers, antipsychotic medications, blood pressure medications, and antihistamines (If you take any of these medications, do not discontinue them without discussing it with your doctor.)
- Being sedentary
- Having vitamin D deficiency
- Experiencing major stress or illness

Factors That Can Improve Insulin Resistance

- Substituting healthy fats for refined carbs
- Eating foods that contain polyphenols (green tea, cocoa, red wine, berries), antioxidants, and omega-3 fatty acids
- Eating such spices as ginger, cinnamon, turmeric, chili pepper, cumin, and oregano
- Choosing fat-free and low-fat dairy products
- Exercising (both cardio and strength training), even if it doesn't lead to weight loss
- Losing weight (especially belly fat)
- Sitting less and taking one- to two-minute walking breaks throughout the day
- Reducing added sugar in your diet
- Practicing stress-reduction techniques

Magnesium Matters

Your body needs magnesium for many reasons, but one that concerns me most for people who are insulin-resistant is its role in the control of blood sugar. In fact, studies suggest that people with higher amounts of magnesium in their bodies have lower rates of type 2 diabetes. Unfortunately, many people don't get enough magnesium in their diets. By making sure you eat magnesium-rich foods (in the amounts specified in the Doctor on Demand plan), you can help your body regulate blood sugar and possibly lower your risk of diabetes.

Top sources of magnesium include:

- Leafy greens
- Nuts and seeds
- Beans and legumes
- Fish
- Whole grains
- Avocados
- Bananas
- Low-fat dairy
- Dark chocolate (hooray!)

What to Do If You're Insulin-Resistant

It's important for you to know whether you are insulin-responsive (which is good) or insulin-resistant (which is not so good) because knowing this can help you customize your Doctor on Demand eating plan in a way that best serves your health and boosts your chances of successful weight loss.

People who are insulin-resistant benefit from being a little more attentive to both the quality and quantity of carbohydrates they ingest. Research shows that for people with insulin resistance, a lower-carb, slightly higher-fat diet (with plenty of lean protein) is generally healthier for them and a more effective way to lose weight.

By making the right choices, you can help decrease your insulin resistance and improve your insulin responsiveness over time. And if you lose weight (especially if you drop inches from your waist), improve your diet, and become more active, you'll have a good shot at lowering your risk of developing prediabetes and type 2 diabetes.

The only way to know for sure if you're insulin-resistant is to be tested by your doctor. However, the following quiz can give you a pretty good idea of whether insulin resistance is an issue for you. If it is, you can use the Customize Your Carbs Plan to tackle insulin resistance head-on.

QUIZ
Insulin Resistance Check-In

Note: If you have been diagnosed with type-2 diabetes, pre-diabetes, or PCOS, you can skip this quiz and assume you're insulin-resistant. If not, answer as many of the questions below as possible:

Do you have high blood pressure (greater than 135/85 mmHg), or are you on blood pressure medication?	yes ☐ no ☐
Do you have high triglycerides (greater than 150 mg/dL) or are you taking medication to lower triglycerides? (Triglycerides are a kind of fat found in the blood.)	yes ☐ no ☐
Do you have low HDL cholesterol (less than 40 mg/dL for men, less than 50 mg/dL for women)?	yes ☐ no ☐
Do you have higher than normal blood sugar or high blood sugar (greater than 100 mg/dL) or are you on a medication such as metformin to lower blood sugar?	yes ☐ no ☐
Is your waist greater than 35 inches if you are a woman or greater than 40 inches if you are a man? *(To measure your waist, pull away clothing and use a flexible tape measure. Starting at the top of your hip bone, wrap the tape measure around your body, keeping it level with your navel and parallel to the floor. Relax your breath and measure.)*	yes ☐ no ☐
Have you started to go through menopause, or are you postmenopausal?	yes ☐ no ☐
Did you have gestational diabetes or a baby heavier than 9 pounds?	yes ☐ no ☐
Do you have a parent or sibling with type 2 diabetes?	yes ☐ no ☐

Do you have a family background that is African American, Alaska Native, American Indian, Asian American, Hispanic/Latino, or Pacific Islander American?	yes ☐ no ☐
Are you very sedentary, meaning you get little or no exercise?	yes ☐ no ☐
Are you under a significant amount of stress? (For example, are you dealing with a very stressful situation in your life, such as unemployment, financial worries, difficult family relationships, a significant health problem, or other major stressors?)	yes ☐ no ☐

Results

- If you answered yes to zero, one, or two of the questions, you have a lower risk of being insulin-resistant. Only your doctor can tell you this for sure, but the risk of insulin resistance is lower for people with few or no risk factors. *I suggest you follow the Insulin-Responsive track of the Customize Your Carbs Plan.*

- If you answered yes to three or more of the questions, you have a higher likelihood of being insulin-resistant. *If this is the case, I recommend that you assume you're insulin-resistant and follow the Insulin-Resistant track of the Customize Your Carbs Plan.*

- If you don't know the answer to all of the questions but answered yes to at least two and consider your body to be apple-shaped and you are a man over 40 or a woman over 50, I recommend that you assume you have some degree of insulin resistance even though the only way to know for sure is to consult a doctor. *For this reason, I advise you to follow the Insulin-Resistant track of the Customize Your Carbs Plan.*

Now that you know which track will suit you best, here's a guide to what foods you can eat in this phase of the Doctor on Demand Diet.

The Customize Your Carbs Plan

The following chart shows you all of the foods included in the Customize Your Carbs Plan. You'll notice that insulin-responsive choices differ somewhat from insulin-resistant choices. People who are insulin-resistant do better (and lose weight faster) if they eat less sugar, fewer carbs, and slightly more fat than those who are insulin-responsive. In a nutshell, here are the differences between the two tracks:

	Insulin-Responsive	Insulin-Resistant
Dense Carbs	Up to 3–4 servings per day	Up to 2–3 servings per day
Fruit	Up to 3 servings per day	Up to 2 servings per day; limit higher-sugar fruit to 1 serving per day and be sure to eat with protein, dairy, or healthy fat. Avoid juice and dried fruit, and limit canned fruit.
Fat	Up to 3–4 servings per day	Up to 5–6 servings per day
Snacks	If you are insulin-resistant, most snacks should contain some form of protein or a healthy fat.	

In addition to allowing you to Customize Your Carbs, this second phase of the Doctor on Demand Diet gives you more foods to choose from. Use the chart below to create your daily meal plans.

Planning Your Customize Your Carbs Meals

You can use the following guide to plan Customize Your Carbs meals. This is the most common way that Doctor on Demand users choose to allocate their proteins, fat, and carbs. You can also use one of the modification options below, or design your own daily eating schedule. Just remember to include protein at all meals and most/all snacks, and to pay especially careful attention to how much fat and how many dense carbs you eat each day.

And don't forget to take a look at the Customize Your Carbs Sample Menu in the back of this book.

Type of Food	
Pure Protein *(Includes low-fat pure protein and higher-fat pure protein)*	**Daily Servings** Women: 8–12 ounces per day (measured after cooking); Men: 10–14 ounces per day *Note: 1 ounce = 7 grams protein*

Sample Foods

Pure Protein

(Includes low-fat pure protein and higher-fat pure protein)

Skinless white-meat poultry

Extra-lean ground white-meat poultry

White fish (flounder, haddock, trout, sole, cod, tilapia)

Shellfish (shrimp, clams, scallops, lobster, imitation crab)

Fresh tuna or canned tuna packed in water

Lean red meat (tenderloin, London broil, top sirloin, choice top round—loin and round are the leanest cuts)

Buffalo

Bison

Low-fat lunch meat (less than 1 gram of fat per ounce)

Eggs/egg whites (1 ounce = 1 whole egg or 2 egg whites)

Protein powder (low-sugar; 7 grams is equivalent to 1 ounce of protein)

Pork (ham, Canadian bacon, tenderloin)

Duck (no skin), ostrich

Higher-Fat Proteins

(*watch portion sizes very carefully and limit to no more than 1–2 servings per week*)

Dark-meat poultry

Salmon*

Ground beef (at least 90% lean)

Higher-fat beef (T-bone, porterhouse, roast, lean ground beef)

Lamb (chop, roast, ground)

Veal (roast, lean chop)

Chicken or turkey sausage

Pork (top loin, chop, cutlet)

Because salmon is loaded with heart-healthy fat, you can consume more than twice a week; just watch your serving sizes.

Type of Food	
Mixed Protein *(Includes starchy protein, fatty protein, dairy protein, vegetarian protein)*	**Daily Servings** Up to 6 servings per day

Sample Foods

Starchy Protein

(limit 2–3 per day if insulin-resistant, 3–4 per day if insulin-responsive; count as **both** *a mixed protein and a dense carb)*

1/2 cup cooked beans

Fatty Protein

(limit 1–2 servings per day if insulin-responsive and 2–3 servings per day if insulin-resistant; count as **both** *a mixed protein and 1 fat)*

2 tablespoons nuts+

1 tablespoon nut butter+

2 tablespoons seeds+

+ *Portion sizes of nuts and seeds are different when counted as protein vs. fat because they contain less protein than fat*

Dairy Protein

(limit 2 per day)

Low-Fat Dairy Protein

6 ounces plain, nonfat yogurt, preferably Greek or Iceland style

1/2 cup fat-free or low-fat cottage cheese

1 ounce low-fat hard cheese or string cheese

1 cup fat-free milk

1.5 ounces low-fat cheese (less than 3 grams fat per serving)

2–3 tablespoons fresh grated Parmesan or part skim mozzarella

1/3 cup low-fat ricotta

Medium-High Fat Dairy Protein

(limit 1 serving per day)

1 ounce full-fat cheese, goat cheese, or mozzarella

2 tablespoons blue cheese or feta

1/4 cup ricotta

Vegetarian Protein

(limit 2 per day unless you are a vegetarian)

1 cup unsweetened soy milk

3 ounces tofu

Type of Food	
Dense Carbs	**Daily Servings** **Insulin-Responsive:** Up to 3–4 servings per day **Insulin-Resistant:** Up to 2–3 servings per day *Notes:* ↝ *If you are smaller, less-active, a women over 50, or have less weight to lose, stay on the lower end of your range.* ↝ *A serving is 80 to 100 calories, and approximately 15 grams of carbohydrates.* ↝ *If you are insulin-resistant, it is especially important to try to eat only whole-grain versions of these foods.* ↝ *If you are not eating gluten, choose gluten-free dense carbs.*

Sample Foods

1/2 cup cooked beans

1/2 cup cooked whole grains, including quinoa, brown rice, barley, etc.

1/2 cup whole-grain cereal (aim for at least 5 grams fiber per serving)

1/2 cup cooked oats (1/4 cup raw)

1/2 cup whole-grain pasta

1/2 cup starchy vegetables, such as corn or peas

1/2 medium or 1/2 cup mashed or baked sweet potato

1/2 medium or 1/2 cup mashed or baked white potato (with skin)

1 slice of whole-grain bread

1 whole-grain sandwich thin

1 small whole-wheat tortilla (100 calories or less)

1 serving whole-grain crackers (approximately 80–100 calories)

1 small corn tortilla

3 cups air-popped popcorn

Type of Food	
Fruit	**Daily Servings** **Insulin-Responsive:** Up to 3 servings per day **Insulin-Resistant:** Up to 2 servings per day *Notes:* ╺ *If you prefer fruit over dense carbs, you may replace 1 dense carb with 1 fruit per day.* ╺ *If you are very active, have more than 50 pounds to lose, or are younger than 50, you may add an additional fruit each day if you find yourself getting very hungry.* ╺ *Canned fruit in water is acceptable in this phase but whole fruit is a much better choice, especially if you are insulin-resistant. Most canned fruit is lower in fiber but still contains water so it is not as calorie-dense as dried fruit. Make sure it is canned in water, not syrup.* ╺ *Serving sizes of canned fruit are slightly smaller than fresh fruit.* ╺ *If you're insulin-resistant, avoid dried fruit and fruit juice.*

Sample Foods

Lower-Sugar Fruit

1 small apple/orange/pear

1/2 grapefruit

1 cup fresh or frozen berries/sliced strawberries or 8 medium whole strawberries

1 medium peach or 1/2 cup frozen chopped peaches

2 apricots

1 large plum

2 fresh tangerines/mandarin oranges/cuties

1 cup melon

1 kiwi

1/2 papaya

Higher-Sugar Fruit

(limit to 1 serving per day if insulin-resistant, and eat with protein, dairy, or healthy fat)

1 small or 1/2 large banana

1/2 mango

1 cup pineapple

1 cup cherries

2 small or 1 large fig

1 cup grapes

Type of Food
Fruit (*continued*)

Sample Foods
Canned Fruit
1/2 cup fruit cocktail
3/4 cup mandarin oranges
1/2 cup canned peaches, pears, or pineapple

Dried fruit
(limit to 1 serving per day if insulin-responsive; avoid if insulin-resistant)
2 tablespoons raisins
3 dried prunes

100% Fruit Juice
(limit as much as possible if insulin-responsive; avoid if insulin-resistant)
4 ounces 100% fruit juice

Non-Starchy Vegetables	**Daily Servings** At least 5 servings per day

Sample Foods
1/2 cup cooked or 1 cup raw fresh or frozen vegetables

Type of Food

Fats	**Daily Servings**
	Insulin-Resistant: 5–6 servings per day
	Insulin-Responsive: 3–4 servings per day
	Notes:
	☙ *A serving is approximately 50 calories, 5 grams of fat.*
	☙ *If you are smaller, less active, older than 50, or have less weight to lose, stay on the low end of the range.*
	☙ *Fats that are higher in saturated fat may contribute to insulin resistance and heart disease and should be limited to 1–2 servings per day.*

Sample Foods

Healthy Fats

1 teaspoon olive or canola oil

1 tablespoon salad dressing or 2 tablespoons low-fat salad dressing (check labels, as calories vary by type of dressing)

8–10 olives

1/4 avocado or 2 tablespoons guacamole

2 tablespoons hummus

1 cup unsweetened almond milk or coconut milk beverage (not coconut milk, which is much higher in calories)

2 tablespoons shredded coconut

1 tablespoon nuts+

1 tablespoon chopped nuts or seeds+

1/2 tablespoon nut butter+

+ *Portion sizes of nuts and seeds are different when counted as protein vs. fat because they contain less protein than fat.*

Fats Higher in Saturated Fat *(limit to 1–2 servings per day)*

1 teaspoon butter

1 teaspoon mayonnaise

1 tablespoon reduced-fat mayo

2 teaspoons whipped butter

2 tablespoons sour cream

3 tablespoons reduced-fat sour cream

2 tablespoons half-and-half (limit, as high in saturated fat)

1 tablespoon cream cheese

2 tablespoons low-fat cream cheese

Beverages	**Daily Servings** Aim for up to 8 cups a day
Unsweetened tea or black coffee (limit caffeinated beverages to 3 servings daily) Water (flat or sparkling, plain or fruit-infused) Sugar-free beverages (limit artificially sweetened drinks as much as possible)	

For a 10-Day Customize Your Carbs Sample Menu, see the Menu section at the back of this book.

The Customize Your Carbs Suggested Daily Meal Plan

Note:

- ❧ If you are *insulin-resistant,* stay on the lower end of the dense carb recommendations for each meal most of the time.
- ❧ If you are *insulin-responsive,* stay on the lower end of the fat recommendations for each meal most of the time.

Breakfast:

- ❧ 1 dairy protein (or 2–3 pure proteins)
- ❧ 1 fruit and/or 1 dense carb
- ❧ 1–2 fats

Lunch:

- ❧ 3–4 proteins (pure protein or combination of pure and mixed protein)
- ❧ 2–3 vegetables
- ❧ 1–2 dense carbs
- ❧ 1–2 fats

Dinner:

- ❧ 3–5 proteins (pure protein or combination of pure and mixed protein)
- ❧ 2–3 vegetables
- ❧ 1–2 dense carbs
- ❧ 1–2 fats

Continues ▶

Full-Size Snack:
- 1 dairy protein (or pure protein or fatty protein)
- PLUS 1 fruit (or dense carb or vegetable)

Mini Snack/Dessert:
- 1 dairy protein (or pure protein or fatty protein)
- OR 1 low-sugar fruit
- OR 1/2 dairy protein + 1/2 to 1 fruit or 1 fat

Or make it your way with any of these modifications:

If you are insulin-resistant:
- Skip dense carbs at any meal to double up at another.
- If you want to add a third snack, cut one fat or protein at lunch or dinner and have with vegetables as a third snack.
- If you want a little fruit with lunch, cut back to half a serving of fruit at breakfast or snack and have the other half with lunch.
- Love nuts? Have two fatty proteins as your full-size snack (1/4 cup nuts) alone or with vegetables only.
- Add a non-starchy vegetable to any meal or snack to make it more satisfying.

If you are insulin-responsive:
- Skip the fat at any meal to double up at another.
- Have fruit with lunch if you limit yourself to one dense carb.
- If you want to add a third snack, cut one dense carb at lunch or dinner and have with one low-fat dairy (just don't exceed your daily dairy total) as a third snack.
- You can have one fruit plus two dense carbs at breakfast as long as you don't exceed four dense carbs per day.
- Add a non-starchy vegetable to any meal or snack to make it more satisfying.

Do You Have Sleep Apnea?

There's one more condition that is worth taking a look at. Sleep apnea is a commonly undiagnosed roadblock to weight loss that is also associated with insulin resistance, and if you have it, you should know about it.

During sleep, people with sleep apnea experience breathing pauses that can last from a few seconds to a minute or longer. These pauses may occur infrequently or as often as 30 or more times per hour. After a pause, normal breathing resumes, sometimes with a choking or snorting sound.

Sleep apnea disrupts sleep and lowers the overall quality of slumber. People with sleep apnea can feel very tired during the day and can have trouble focusing on everyday tasks.

Being overweight increases your risk of sleep apnea, because excess fat tissue in the neck area can make it harder to breathe. But the connection goes the other way, too: if you're trying to lose weight, having sleep apnea can make weight loss more difficult, because being exhausted during the day makes it harder to stay committed to a diet and exercise plan. What's more, inadequate sleep can alter your hunger and satiety hormones in a way that makes you want more food and feel less satisfied after you eat. Even if you don't have sleep apnea, it's important to get enough rest every night.

One of the problems with sleep apnea is that many people are unaware that they have it. That's why identifying sleep apnea, and then getting treatment for it, can take away a big obstacle to weight loss. I've had many patients who, after struggling unsuccessfully to lose weight, discovered they had undiagnosed sleep apnea. Once they started treatment for the condition, they were able to lose weight. (Sleep apnea is treated with life-style changes, breathing devices, mouthpieces, and in extreme cases, surgery.) When people with sleep apnea lose weight, their condition typically improves—in fact, significant weight loss in an obese person can make sleep apnea disappear.

Only a doctor or other health-care provider can definitively diagnose sleep apnea. However, the following assessment can help you determine whether you are at higher risk of having the condition. The following questions are based on what's referred to as the "STOP-BANG" Questionnaire that some health-care providers use to diagnose sleep apnea.

Sleep Apnea Questionnaire

Do you snore loudly (louder than talking or loud enough to be heard through closed doors)?	yes ☐ no ☐
Do you often feel tired, fatigued, or sleepy during daytime?	yes ☐ no ☐
Has anyone observed you stop breathing during your sleep?	yes ☐ no ☐
Do you have or are you being treated for high blood pressure?	yes ☐ no ☐
Is your BMI more than 35?	yes ☐ no ☐
Are you over 50 years old?	yes ☐ no ☐
Is your neck circumference greater than 17 inches if you're a man or 16 inches if you're a woman?	yes ☐ no ☐
Are you male?	yes ☐ no ☐

Results:

- If you answered yes to three or more questions, your risk of sleep apnea is higher. It's definitely worthwhile to follow up with a health care professional. If you have sleep apnea, your provider can offer the treatment you need to sleep more soundly, which may pave the way for more successful weight loss as well.

- If you answered yes to fewer than three questions, your risk of sleep apnea is lower. Even so, if you are concerned, you may want to follow up with your doctor.

Adapted from "STOP Questionnaire: A Tool to Screen Patients for Obstructive Sleep Apnea." Frances Chung, FRCPC, Balaji Yegneswaran, MBBS, Pu Liao, MD, Sharon A. Chung, PhD, Santhira Vairavanathan, MBBS, Sazzadul Islam, MSc, Ali Khajehdehi, MD, Colin M. Shapiro, FRCPC, *Anesthesiology* 2008; 108:812–21 Copyright © 2008, the American Society of Anesthesiologists, Inc., Lippincott Williams & Wilkins, Inc.

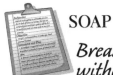

SOAP Notes

Breast Cancer Survivor Loses Weight without Feeling Deprived

Cynthia is a 57-year-old woman with a history of breast cancer, high cholesterol, prediabetes, and an underactive thyroid. She had lost weight in the past with a commercial weight-loss program, but after her breast cancer treatment she found that what worked previously was no longer effective for her. She needed to lose only 15 pounds and she was not in a rush—she wanted a livable strategy and loved to cook, and she didn't want to feel deprived or bored. This note reflects her first 10 days on my program.

Subjective:

Patient reports decreased appetite with reduced dense carb intake, but misses having pasta dinners. Is doing interval training twice a week, and feels a real difference in how hard she is able to work out. She is not doing weight training yet, because she does not belong to a gym. She occasionally gets very hungry at lunch or midafternoon.

Objective:

Down 3.4 pounds. Food journal shows inadequate protein at breakfast on days when she is very hungry at lunch, and no dense carbs at lunch when she is hungry in the afternoon.

Assessment and Plan:

1. Breakfast: Be more consistent with morning protein, because it helps curb hunger in early part of day. I recommended a cookbook with interesting recipes, since she enjoys cooking.

2. Lunch: Make sure to include a dense carb at lunch to satisfy hunger, and make sure to plan ahead for a protein-based midafternoon snack that she should eat *before* she becomes hungry, such as yogurt with berries or a snack-size breakfast smoothie.

3. Timing: Suggested patient skip two cycling days [*more about this in the next chapter*] in Phase 3 unless she hits a weight-loss plateau, since she is not in a rush to lose weight and really enjoys and feels satisfied by having dense carbs with most meals.

The Facts about Sugar Substitutes

Artificial sweeteners, including saccharin, aspartame, acesulfame-K, and sucralose, are the most commonly used sugar substitutes. They are considered food additives and have essentially no calories. All are considered safe, according to the US Food and Drug Administration (FDA). Their role in weight loss is somewhat controversial, but a recent meta-analysis suggests that when they are used in place of sugar, they can help modestly with weight loss and may improve compliance with weight-loss and weight-maintenance plans.

Some research suggests that artificial sweeteners may adversely affect gut bacteria and increase cravings for sugar, but the clinical significance of these findings has not been established.

In my opinion, based on current research, artificial sweeteners are okay to use in moderation. I don't think it's a good idea to rely heavily on them, but if using them once in a while helps you eat healthy foods—for example, Greek yogurt—then I think they're fine for occasional use.

Another kind of sugar substitute is sugar alcohols, including sorbitol, mannitol, xylitol, erythritol, lactitol, and maltitol. These are commercially produced sweeteners that offer several advantages over sugar. They have less of an impact on blood sugar, and because they are not absorbed completely by the body, they have fewer calories per gram than regular sugar, so they can be helpful for weight and blood sugar control. However, because they are not fully absorbed by the body, excess consumption can lead to gas and diarrhea.

My top choice for a sugar substitute is stevia, a natural, no-calorie sweetener made from a South American plant. Highly purified stevia extract, which is the version found on the market, is considered safe by the FDA, and some evidence suggests that it may actually improve blood sugar control. I use a stevia sweetener packet in my coffee every morning and to sweeten my plain Greek yogurt and low-fat ricotta for dessert recipes. I also drink a soda sweetened with stevia on occasion.

4. Weight training: Recommended simple home weight routine with exercise bands. Encouraged patient to purchase exercise class trial packages at local gyms using daily discount websites that would allow her to try out a variety of options and eventually find something that she would enjoy and do long term.

Result:

Cynthia lost the 15 pounds in four months. Both she and I were surprised at how easily and steadily the weight came off.

—*Melina B. Jampolis, MD*

 Clinical Pearl: *Raising the Bar*

I have to admit, I'm a big fan of energy bars as a quick snack or on-the-go breakfast, especially when I'm travelling. Yes, real food is always the healthiest choice, but this diet is about being practical, not perfect. Most energy bars are loaded with sugar, calories, and saturated fat. If you enjoy energy bars on occasion, you can reintroduce them during this phase. Aim for bars that have *no more than* 200 calories, 12 grams of sugar or less, 5 grams of fat or less, at least 3 grams of fiber, and at least 10 grams of protein. Consider them one dense carb, one fat, and one to two lean proteins. Even though they are often labeled "all natural," I'm not a huge fan of the fruit and nut bars for weight loss because both nuts and dried fruit are very calorie dense, so you consume a lot of calories but not a lot of volume or protein for optimal hunger control. If you choose these types of bars, count them as one fat protein, one fat, and one fruit.

Coming Up Next: Cycle for Success

Once you complete Phase 2 and learn how to Customize Your Carbs, you'll be ready to move on to Phase 3 of the Doctor on Demand Diet—the Cycle for Success Plan. In this phase, I'll explain how a process called Diet-Cycling can help you reach your weight-loss goal and maintain your healthy weight for the rest of your life, while giving you even more flexibility and choice to enjoy delicious, nutritious meals.

CHAPTER 3

—⟋ɷ⟍—

Phase 3:
The Cycle for Success Plan

Welcome to Phase 3 of the Doctor on Demand Diet. In this third and final phase, the Cycle for Success Plan, we'll be focusing on two main goals:

- Prevent plateaus, which can be very discouraging and often cause people to abandon their weight-loss plan.
- Build even more flexibility into your daily and weekly food choices if you need it and want it.

We'll address these two very important objectives with a strategy called Diet-Cycling, which can be an incredibly effective way to lose weight while still enjoying your food and not feeling deprived.

By now you should be seeing some impressive results, including weight loss of anywhere from 5 to 10 pounds, increased energy, better insulin responsiveness (you can't actually see this, but you can be fairly certain it's happening), and the strong sense of satisfaction you get from a job well done and building a solid foundation for lasting weight loss.

If you don't feel ready to move on to the Cycle for Success Plan, feel free to hold off. You can choose to repeat the CleanStart Plan (Phase 1) or the Customize Your Carbs Plan (Phase 2) for another 10 days. Or, give Cycle for Success a spin and see how you do with it.

Remember, the underlying objective of the Doctor on Demand program is "structured flexibility." All three plans offer you both structure *and* flexibility, but as you progress from Phase 1 to Phase 2 to Phase 3, structure decreases and flexibility increases. If you crave structure more than flexibility, staying with an earlier phase may work best for you.

Cycling for Flexibility

I focus on flexibility in the Cycle for Success Plan because, having spent the last 14 years helping patients to lose weight, I know that the same approach does not work for everyone. I've found that success is more likely when we can customize a plan to take into account our own individual lifestyle, health, and preferences. I've also learned that for people who live busy lives—which, after all, is most of us—having a flexible eating plan can really help fit your diet into your everyday life.

Our goal in this phase is to develop an approach that truly works for you now and for the weeks, months, and years to come as you continue to lose weight, reach your goal weight, and maintain your weight loss long-term.

I recommend Diet-Cycling during this phase because it makes continued weight loss more livable. Research shows that most people can't stay on extreme diets (very low-carb, low-fat, or low-calorie) for the long term. Generally, people on difficult-to-follow diets invariably end up migrating away from their strenuous eating regimens, which can cause discouragement and often slows or reverses weight loss.

The same is true of my patients. Having to stick with a challenging plan every single day of the week (including weekends) can be difficult, and for some people, it can be too much to deal with. But when they can alternate easier days with more challenging days, they do much better over time.

I learned this through trial and error with my patients and myself. I noticed that many people with large amounts of weight to lose did fine at first—they could cut back on calories, fat, and carbs successfully for several weeks. But over time, they started to develop a kind of diet fatigue. I knew they had to stick with their plans in order to support ongoing weight loss, but I also knew that they needed some help. So rather than asking my patients to cut calories, fat, and carbs significantly from their diets seven days a week, I started asking them to do so for just two days a week while following a more moderate plan the other five days. This strategy of "Diet-Cycling"—going back and forth between more challenging and less challenging daily eating plans—worked out really well.

When my patients Diet-Cycle, they are much more successful in sticking with the program long-term. They also maintain a higher level of motivation because of the sustained rate of weight loss they experience and the fact that they don't have to keep continuously reducing calories (and risking the feeling of deprivation) in order to keep losing weight.

A Modified Approach

My Diet-Cycling strategy was sparked in part by research suggesting that a strategy known as alternate-day modified fasting (ADMF) may help improve insulin resistance and facilitate weight loss.

ADMF generally involves restricting calories to 500 per day on modified fasting days, which I think is incredibly difficult for most people. I asked myself if I could limit myself to 500 calories several days a week, and the answer was a resolute NO. But the concept behind ADMF intrigued me, so I customized a plan based on ADMF that was far less stringent but still very effective.

I created two different kinds of cycling days—one for people who are insulin-responsive, and one for people who are insulin-resistant. Once I tweaked it and determined that it worked well for several patients, I started recommending my Cycle for Success Plan to most of my patients. I've been very impressed with the results, and I think you will be, too.

Cycling is especially helpful for people who have difficulty sticking to their weight-loss programs on weekends. In general, weekends tend to be less structured when it comes to eating and exercise, and they typically involve more social eating occasions. Using the Cycle for Success Plan, you can relax a bit on weekends and focus more on cutting calories, carbs, and fat during the week, when it's less of a challenge.

Although some research shows that people who are most consistent with their eating on weekdays and weekends tend to be more successful at weight loss, I find that this approach is not realistic for most of my patients, particularly if they have active social lives, travel often, or have a lot of weight to lose (meaning they are going to be following this diet for a long time).

In addition, unless you have only 10 to 15 pounds to lose, you will inevitably have to face holidays and social eating situations where you may not be entirely in control of what you are served (in addition to having to continuously resist temptations like wine or apple pie or birthday cake). I like to think of the two-day-per-week "Clean Days" as an instant autocorrect for your diet to keep you on track.

Designing Your Own Cycle for Success Plan

Following the Cycle for Success Plan is easy. In a nutshell, here's what you do:

If you are insulin-responsive, continue to use the Customize Your Carbs Plan that you followed in Phase 2 for *five* days a week. Then, for *two* days a week (your "Clean Days"), follow the Phase 1 CleanStart Plan, which requires you to cut back down to two dense carbs (and no dry carbs) and three fats per day.

By switching back to the CleanStart Plan for two days, you're lowering your daily intake of calories, carbohydrates, and fat. This helps you jump-start your weight loss and push through plateaus. But because you continue to eat healthy amounts of protein at meals and snacks, you keep your metabolism humming. And by choosing foods that make every calorie count, you help maximize weight loss and minimize hunger. You also have the option of following the insulin-resistant plan explained below, which some of my patients find simpler.

If you are insulin-resistant, continue to use the Customize Your Carbs Plan that you followed in Phase 2 for *five* days a week. Then, for *two* days a week (your "Clean Days"), follow the Customize Your Carbs Plan with one change: eliminate all dense carbs for the day.

By taking the simple step of eliminating all dense carbs two days a week, you cut calories while also taking a lower-carbohydrate approach that helps improve insulin resistance. Although calories are lower, you continue to eat healthy amounts of protein and fat at meals and snacks. And by cutting dense carbs rather than vegetables or fruits, you lower your carbohydrate intake without cheating yourself of the many valuable nutrients found in carbohydrate foods.

A Plan for Life

You can continue following the Cycle for Success Plan for the rest of your life. As you go along, you can modify it to fit your weight and your life. For example, when you hit a plateau, you can add a third day of cycling to your week until you break through. And when you reach your goal weight, you can experiment with the Cycle for Success Plan to figure out the best way to maintain your weight loss. You may decide to Diet-Cycle only one day a week. Or you may only need to Diet-Cycle if you put on a pound or two. It's your choice.

For a 10-Day Cycle for Success Sample Menu, see the Menu section at the back of this book.

Sample Insulin-Resistant Cycle Day (No Dense Carbs)

Breakfast:
- 1 dairy protein (or 2–3 pure proteins)
- 1 fruit
- 1–2 fats

Lunch:
- 3–4 proteins (pure protein or combination of pure and mixed protein)
- 2–3 vegetables
- 1–2 fats

Dinner:
- 4–5 proteins (pure protein or combination of pure and mixed protein)
- 2–3 vegetables
- 1–2 fats

Full-Size Snack:
- 1 dairy protein (or pure protein or fatty protein)
- PLUS 1 fruit or vegetable

Mini Snack/Dessert:
- 1 dairy protein (or pure protein or fatty protein)
- OR 1/2 dairy + 1/2 fruit or 1 fat

*If you can't live without dense carbs, even just for a day, you can include 1 dense carb from the CleanStart phase (no bread).

Sample Insulin-Resistant Cycle Day (No Dense Carbs)

Breakfast:
- 1 dairy protein (or 2–3 pure proteins)
- 1 fruit
- 1–2 fats

Lunch:
- 3–4 proteins (pure protein or combination of pure and mixed protein)
- 2–3 vegetables
- 1–2 fats

Dinner:
- 4–5 proteins (pure protein or combination of pure and mixed protein)
- 2–3 vegetables
- 1–2 fats

Full Size Snack:
- 1 dairy protein (or pure protein or fatty protein)
- PLUS 1 fruit or vegetable

Mini Snack/Dessert:
- 1 dairy protein (or pure protein or fatty protein)
- OR 1/2 dairy + 1/2 fruit *or* 1 fat

*If you can't live without dense carbs, even just for a day, you can include 1 dense carb from the CleanStart phase (no bread).

Which days of the week are best for cycling? That's up to you. Many of my patients find that the best choice for them is to Diet-Cycle on Mondays and Wednesdays. That allows them to make a fresh start early in the week and to make up for any weekend splurges. In addition, they find it preferable not to schedule cycling days back-to-back, because that helps maintain optimal energy levels and minimize carbohydrate cravings. Other patients prefer to get their cycling days out of the way right up front by cycling on Mondays and Tuesday, and some find it easier to Diet-Cycle on weekends when they have more control over all of their meals and can really focus on making lower-calorie or lower-carbohydrate meals taste terrific.

You also have the option of cycling more often—or less often—than two days a week. Cycling more often will help speed up weight loss. Cycling less often will slow it down, but for some people, that slower pace is just right.

And of course, you have the option of cycling back and forth among all three phases whenever you want. Remember, the goal is to find the strategies that best allow you to lose weight now and for all of the weeks or months it takes for you to get to your goal weight. If a slow-but-steady approach works better for you than the fast track, then by all means, do what works best for you.

Even More Flexibility with Flex Blocks

In addition to using Diet-Cycling as a way to give you more flexibility, the Cycle for Success Plan offers you the option of using Flex Blocks. These allow you to eat controlled portions of foods and drinks you may miss, such as sweets and alcohol. Flex Blocks allow you to enjoy a few treats without totally blowing your program, and are designed to make this plan more livable and to start teaching you how to build in more indulgent foods long-term. (Who can avoid cocktails and cookies forever? I know I can't!)

You don't have to use your Flex Blocks. If you can stay focused without them, your progress will be faster. If you don't want to deal with any temptation or feel that you want to lose more weight before indulging, no problem. But I've found with my patients that it's better to have occasional controlled portions of "treat" foods once in a while than to attempt to cut them out of your life forever. Indulging in occasional Flex Block foods allows you to have a bit of something you crave and still stay on track rather than letting a feeling of deprivation push you off your weight-loss plan completely.

Like so many of the other strategies in this book, Flex Blocks are tools that you should use when you need them and set aside when you don't.

Here's how Flex Blocks work. Each week, you can incorporate up to five Flex Blocks into your eating plan if you Diet-Cycle for two days per week. (If you Diet-Cycle for only one day, cut Flex Blocks down to two or three a week.) Flex Blocks can be used on the weekends or anytime during the week that you need a treat (or a glass of wine). The only days you shouldn't use Flex Blocks are Clean Days—days on which you are cycling—since those days are purposely lower in calories and carbohydrates.

If necessary—say if you're attending a wedding or special party and really want to splurge—you can use up to three Flex Blocks at one time. But overall it's best to use one at a time. And if you don't use them, you can't "bank" them for the next week. Remember, they are tools to help you stick with your weight-loss plan long-term.

The 411 on Flex Blocks

Flexibility is the name of the game, so use the Flex Blocks only if you need them and try your best to plan ahead for their use. Be very careful that they don't exceed the weekly total if you are still trying to actively lose weight. I also recommend that you avoid spending your Flex Blocks on "trigger" foods (foods that trigger overeating) as much as possible and be very diligent about portion sizes to keep calories under control.

Adding Flex Blocks can be a problem for some people. Quite a few of my patients have an all-or-nothing mentality—they either eat perfectly or go off the program completely. If you're an all-or-nothing type, you may not want to use Flex Blocks.

In general, it's up to you to decide whether and when to use Flex Blocks. I find that the most successful patients are those who are able to include occasional indulgent foods (or beverages) into their diet without going off track. Since I'm not seeing you as a patient, however, I can't help fine-tune this aspect of your diet for you—you'll have to find your own best balance. Don't worry, you can do it: for most people, a little trial and error shows exactly what works best for you. If you're not using a food journal, reconsider giving it a try. Writing down everything you eat (when, what, and how much) will help you determine the best way to use your Flex Blocks and will allow you to determine whether they are beneficial to you. If your food journal suggests that Flex Blocks are not helpful, you don't have to use them.

Flex Block Choices

- **Alcohol:** 5 ounces of wine, 12 ounces light beer, 1.5 ounces spirits (plain or mixed with club soda or seltzer, not juice or sugar syrup). *Note: I strongly recommend limiting alcoholic beverages to a maximum of three servings per week, especially for women.*

The Same Old, Same Old

Is it OK to eat the same foods every day? That's a question many of my patients ask me. The answer depends on *what* you are eating every day.

Many of my patients seem to do better when they stick to a routine during the week and get a bit more variety on weekends. As long as you are focusing on the basic nutrition principles and eating enough fruits and vegetables, you are probably OK. In fact, research shows that people with less variety in their diet seem to do better with weight loss and maintenance.

One of my most successful patients used to chart out his meals for the week every Sunday night. He rotated through the same meals over and over, and yet he never seemed to get bored. He deviated occasionally during the holidays and for things like poker night with the boys or dinner out. It worked for him: he lost 46 pounds in six months and now has the cholesterol and physique of a man 20 years younger.

Personally, I find it much easier in terms of shopping and cooking to stick with just a few different choices for each meal and snack, with small variations (like changing up the protein, nut, grain, fruit, or vegetable). You can do this easily using the meal templates and recipes provided at the end of the book.

- **Dark chocolate:** Up to 1 ounce (approximately 100–150 calories).

- **Reduced-sugar/reduced-fat desserts:** One serving (100–150 calories per serving). Choose a packaged brand, or see the Recipe section for healthier, more satisfying options.

- **Other choices:** I realize that the longer you stay on this diet, the more you may require a wider variety of Flex Block choices. However, I think it's best not to give you a long list of options, because that might imply that I am encouraging you to eat a lot of unhealthy foods. Plus, research shows that the more choices people have for unhealthy foods, the more likely they are to consume more calories. Instead, let's keep it simple: if there are other foods that you generally should avoid (like pancakes, ice cream, cookies, and cakes, to name a few), simply figure out how many calories they contain and have a portion size that's 100 to 150 calories. If you need help with this, consider consulting with a registered dietitian or nutritionist.

SOAP Notes

Losing Weight While Wining and Dining

Carlos is a super-busy TV executive with young children who is on the road several months a year. His doctor referred him to me to manage his prediabetes; he was also being treated for an underactive thyroid and high blood pressure. This note is from a visit about a month into his program, when he had lost only a few pounds.

Subjective:

Patient is exercising only once a week due to his busy travel schedule and his desire to spend time with his children on weekends rather than going to the gym. He also spends a lot of time on workdays sitting and editing TV footage. He drinks wine most nights and eats out on weekends; in restaurants, he is not always careful with fat, bread, and sugar. He also finds it hard to follow his eating plan on the road.

Objective:

Weight down 0.5 pound. Not keeping food journal.

Assessment and Plan:

1. Gluten intake: Because of his history of hypothyroidism, I suggested patient try going off wheat and gluten completely for two weeks.

2. Weekend eating: Cycle in two low-carb (insulin-resistant) days per week to balance out wine and more indulgent weekend eating. I also suggested that if he is going to have more than one glass of wine at dinner, he avoid having any dense carbs at dinner and focus just on having lean protein and vegetables.

3. Travel challenges: I suggested that patient travel with shaker bottle and packets of protein powder for quick, easy, high-protein breakfast or snack on the road.

4. Exercise: If staying at a hotel with a gym, try to squeeze in one or two super-quick interval training sessions when possible—even just 15 minutes can make a difference. During the day, try to get up every hour and walk or stretch for a few minutes. On weekends, exercise in the morning before children wake up to leave plenty of family time later in the day, or plan active family outings that everyone can enjoy.

Result:

After this visit, Carlos lost 4.2 pounds in 11 days. Overall he lost 21 pounds in 5½ months and moved his blood sugar into the normal range. After giving up gluten for two weeks and then reintroducing it, he noticed a big difference in how he felt, so he decided to do his best to stay off gluten as much as possible.

—*Melina B. Jampolis, MD*

Coming Up Next

Congratulations! You've learned everything there is to know about how to use the Doctor on Demand Diet on a day-to-day basis. You've mastered the basics in the CleanStart Plan, fine-tuned your diet based on your body's reaction to carbohydrates in the Customize Your Carbs Plan, and optimized your diet for long-term results and flexibility in the Cycle for Success Plan.

Here's a summary of the three phases of the Doctor on Demand Diet:

Phase 1: CleanStart

- No alcohol, added sugar, or dry carbs (bread, pasta, crackers) for 10 days
- Two dense carbs (starchy vegetable, whole grain, beans) per day
- Protein with every meal and most snacks
- Three fats per day
- Unlimited non-starchy vegetables
- Two low-sugar fruits per day

Phase 2: Customize Your Carbs for Insulin Resistance and Responsiveness

- ᴥ Insulin-responsive: Three to four dense carbs per day; three to four fats per day
- ᴥ Insulin-resistant: Two to three dense carbs per day; five to six fats per day
- ᴥ Protein with every meal and most snacks
- ᴥ No alcohol, limit added sugar
- ᴥ Unlimited non-starchy vegetables
- ᴥ Two fruits per day (insulin-resistant); three fruits per day (insulin-responsive)

Phase 3: Cycle for Success

- ᴥ Follow the Customize your Carbs plan five days per week
- ᴥ Cycle two "clean" days per week: go back to CleanStart or cut dense carbs
- ᴥ Introduce Flex Blocks: Alcoholic beverage or small dessert, up to five servings per week

Now it's time to move on to the non-dietary aspects of the Doctor on Demand Diet. The first is goal setting. In the next chapter, I'll show you how goal setting can be an incredibly helpful tool for you, and how using my goal-setting worksheets can help you formulate, commit to, and achieve goals. In the chapters that follow, I'll give you lots of great info and advice on making great behavior choices, creating a supportive environment, and following your successful program in restaurants and while traveling. We'll also take a look at your exercise preferences and work with those to build a realistic fitness program that's right for you. Finally, I'll give you a game plan that will help you maintain your weight loss indefinitely.

—ᴡ—

Fire Up Your Future
with Goals That Deliver

Now that you understand the food choices I recommend in the Doctor on Demand Diet, it's time to focus on the behavior choices that contribute to successful weight loss. As you do this, it's important to remember that eating behaviors are choices, and no matter how ingrained a behavior is, it's still a choice. Setting realistic goals is one of those behaviors.

Goal setting helps you stay focused, gives you something to shoot for, and provides you with a way to measure success. I encourage my patients to have several types of goals, because they serve different purposes and offer various kinds of motivation. People who succeed tend to have a combination of big goals and small goals, shorter-term goals and longer-term goals.

Although getting down to a particular weight is one kind of goal, overall your goals must go beyond just numbers on a scale. Focusing too much on pounds lost can prevent you from achieving positive results that propel you forward, because some days the number doesn't change—or it changes for the worse. But if you have a range of goals, you can feel a sense of accomplishment even when you face small setbacks.

In this chapter, we'll look at different kinds of weight-loss goals, and I'll give you information and advice on how to set achievable goals. I'll also provide some handy goal-setting worksheets that will help you zero in on which goals are best—and most realistic—for you.

Your goals must be realistic in order to be effective. Expecting too much is a recipe for failure: I've seen too many people give up on weight-loss plans because of unrealistic expectations. They set an unreachable goal and then become disappointed and disillusioned when they don't lose the pounds quickly enough, or when they hit a plateau that is far from their goal weight.

It comes down to understanding *your* reality. How much and how fast you can lose weight is very individual—one person can shed pounds quickly and get to her goal in weeks; the next loses slowly and takes months or even years to get to where he wants to go. What matters is that you know what's realistic for you; otherwise you risk feeling devastated or beating yourself up when you "fail" to meet a goal. When it comes to the rate and amount of weight loss you're aiming for, you're really best off if you respect your own individual reality.

 Clinical Pearl: *Think SMART*

When it comes to setting goals, I want you to think SMART: Specific, Measurable, Attainable, Realistic, and Timely. Setting specific, realistic exercise goals can be a terrific exercise motivator. Goals can be short-term (walk four times this week), medium-term (go to a yoga class every Wednesday for the next month), or longer-term (run a 10K race within six months). Whatever goals you choose, just make sure they are realistic—for example, if you've never run a mile it may be too much to aim to run a 10K or even 5K next month. If you aren't a morning person, don't commit to a 5:00 a.m. boot camp for the next six weeks. Write down your doable goals, commit to them, and make step-by-step plans to achieve them. When you meet goals, celebrate with a reward that doesn't involve food, and then set some new goals that will challenge you even more. ◇

Getting Real with Goals: How Much and How Fast

First let's consider your rate of weight loss. One of the biggest issues I face with my patients on a regular basis is helping them to determine a weight-loss rate that is both appropriate and realistic. If you want to lose 20 pounds in the next month, that's not realistic. Life is not a reality TV show, where you can quit your job, exercise for endless hours each day, and eat food prepared by a personal chef trained to cook the healthiest of foods. In real life, we don't have the luxury of focusing on nothing but losing weight. It's not realistic to expect

Scale Stats

- 68.8 percent of adults are overweight or obese
- 35.7 percent of adults are obese
- 6.3 percent of adults are considered extremely obese (BMI of 40+)
- 33.2 percent of children and adolescents ages 6 to 19 are overweight or obese
- 18.2 percent of children and adolescents ages 6 to 19 are obese

Source: National Institute of Diabetes and Digestive and Kidney Diseases (NIDDK), http://win.niddk.nih.gov/statistics/index.htm

to lose weight that quickly. Even if you could, it wouldn't be good for you (unless you were under the care of an experienced bariatric care physician) because you would lose a significant amount of muscle and bone.

The truth is that it is difficult and not particularly healthy for women to lose more than one to two pounds of fat per week and for men to lose more than two to three pounds of fat per week. So I encourage you to keep those numbers in mind as you think about your weight-loss rate goals.

As for goal weight, a dose of realism helps a lot. If you are hoping to get down to the weight you were in high school—before you had three kids, a mortgage, and a full-time job—you may want to reevaluate. Your body and your life have changed drastically since you were a teenager. Do you really have the time or energy at this point in your life to whittle yourself down to your adolescent weight? Is it worth the sacrifices? For many of us, the answer is no.

For some people, especially younger men, weight loss may not be that difficult. But for most of us the realities of life, such as children, travel, work, sick parents or spouses, and even our genetics, require us to set more realistic goals.

It is also good to remember that metabolism slows down as we age. Loss of muscle mass contributes to this, although some of that is preventable through strength training. But a certain amount of muscle loss is simply the result of aging and normal physical changes in the body, both of which are not within your control. So you do need to factor age into your goal setting, too.

Ask Yourself: What's Comfortable? What's Maintainable?

Another way to choose a weight-loss goal is to choose a weight (or clothing size) that you feel you can achieve and comfortably maintain. Look back at the various weights you've been, and try to remember a weight or size that made you feel comfortable and that you could maintain without a huge struggle. I tend to encourage my patients to focus more on clothing size rather than weight, because healthy changes in body composition (increased muscle-to-fat ratio) can actually increase your weight slightly, while still allowing your pant size to decrease. And gaining muscle shouldn't ever be thought of as a bad thing, because it increases metabolism and helps with overall health as well as weight loss.

After setting your weight-loss goals, you might want to share them with a family member, close friend, or even your physician. Doing this may help you stay on track or give you the added motivation you need to succeed. (Or it may not—it's up to you.)

If you prefer, you don't have to choose a goal weight. It is fine to begin your weight-loss program simply with a goal of losing an as-yet-to-be-defined amount of weight. Your goal can be to fit into a specific pair of pants, or just to become healthier and more active.

If you are not really focused on weight but rather on health, defining health-related goals may work just as well or even better than picking a goal weight. For example, your goals could be to lower your cholesterol level, reduce your blood sugar readings, start exercising every day, or even just to feel less winded when you climb a flight of stairs.

Try Five at a Time

If you need to lose 30 pounds or more, I recommend that you consider setting several smaller weight-loss goals. Start with a goal of 5 percent of your body weight, because this small amount can have a big impact on your long-term health.

Research shows that even among obese people, losing 5 to 10 percent of body weight can have major positive health benefits. For someone who weighs 200 pounds, that's a weight loss of 10 to 20 pounds—which is a very realistic, attainable goal. A modest loss may not get you into the jeans you wore in high school, but it can provide some of the following boosts to your health:

- ↝ An increase in HDL cholesterol (the "good" cholesterol)
- ↝ A drop in triglycerides (a kind of "bad" cholesterol)
- ↝ Lower blood pressure
- ↝ A reduced risk of type 2 diabetes
- ↝ Increased sensitivity to insulin
- ↝ Less inflammation throughout your body
- ↝ Improvement in sleep apnea symptoms

Sure, it would be nice to slim down to a small size. But for people with a lot of weight to lose, the thought of having to lose a large amount of weight can be overwhelming. So instead of setting hard-to-reach goals, consider aiming for that 5 percent drop, because even modest weight loss can go a long way toward improving your health.

Once you have attained your 5 percent goal, reconsider the situation and decide whether you should set a second 5 percent weight-loss goal. Consider a few things: How do you feel? How is your health? How hard was it for you to reach your first goal? Do you still want to lose more, or do you feel better maintaining this weight for a period of time?

Need help figuring out what your 5 to 10 percent weight loss would be? There's a handy worksheet on the next page to guide you.

SOAP Notes
Busy Mom Wants to Lose Baby Weight

Jody is a mom in her mid-30s with young children and excess weight that she never managed to shed after her pregnancies. She had no major medical problems and exercised regularly—spinning twice a week, doing Pilates twice a week, and working out with a personal trainer once a week. Her diet was fairly typical for many of the moms I see with young children: cereal or waffles for breakfast; sandwich or salad for lunch; coffee and a sweet snack or fruit and nut bar with the kids after school; and a relatively balanced, kid-friendly dinner, indulging in a glass of wine and/or dessert several

Doctor on Demand Worksheet:
Determine Your 5 to 10 Percent Weight-Loss Goal

If you have a lot of weight to lose, you may want to start by setting a goal of losing 5 to 10 percent of your body weight. You may ultimately want to lose more than that, but it's a great place to start because it can deliver some fantastic health benefits. To determine your 5 to 10 percent first-step weight-loss goal, fill out the following worksheet:

Your starting weight: _____

Determine your 5% weight loss: Multiply your weight by .95 (your weight minus 5%).

Starting Weight: _____ x .95 = _____

This is the *low end* of your first-step goal weight.

Determine your 10% weight loss: Multiply your weight by .90 (your weight minus 10%).

Starting Weight: _____ x .90 = _____

This is the *high end* of your first-step goal weight.

Fill in: Your first-step goal weight is _____ to _____ pounds.

Once you reach your first-step goal weight, go back and fill out this worksheet again. You may find that rather than lose more weight, you'll simply want to maintain your new weight for a while. Or you may want to keep going. If so, consider setting another 5 to 10 percent goal. By losing weight in steps, you are more likely to succeed. Use the body mass index (BMI) chart on page 100 to help determine a final goal, or for a more personalized recommendation, consult a dietitian or nutritionist.

times a week. This note is from one of her visits about halfway through her program.

Subjective:

Patient feels much better with reduced sugar intake but still needs a treat on a regular basis. Feels much less tired with protein added to afternoon snack. Still snacking on dry carbs in the afternoon while working at her computer, but trying to pay more attention to that. Also, she is trying not to finish uneaten food on her kids' plates. PMS last week led to a couple of "really bad" eating days. With the addition of two days of cardio per week (running or walk/run) and occasional weekend family hikes, she is now reaching the goal of five days of cardio per week.

Objective:

Weight down 1.6 pounds over the previous two weeks. Food journal still shows too many dry-carb snacks such as pretzels, crackers, and kettle corn. Occasionally snacks on handful of trail mix in the evening.

Assessment and Plan:

1. Dry carbs: Cut back on dry carbs and choose either dessert OR wine for daily indulgence.

2. Evening snack: Cut out trail mix, which is high in carbohydrates and calories and lower in protein; have fresh fruit and a small serving of nuts instead.

3. Extra calories: Stop finishing food on kids' plates or in snack bowls— this mindless eating can add several hundred calories per day and can be the difference between losing or gaining a pound or more per week.

4. That time of the month: Don't try to endure cravings when suffering from PMS; if you want chocolate, have chocolate (in a limited amount), and cut back slightly on something else.

Result:

Jody lost 15 pounds over the course of four months and wanted to lose another five, but stopped coming to see me.

—Melina B. Jampolis, MD

Other Ways to Set Weight Goals

Another way to choose a goal weight is by using your body mass index (BMI) as a guide. BMI is a ratio of your height to your weight. A BMI of below 25 is considered "normal" weight; 25 to 29 is overweight; and greater than 30 is obese. The medical community uses BMI as a measure of obesity in research and general practice.

The problem with BMI is that it does not distinguish between lean body mass (muscle, water, bone) and fat mass. For example, a muscular woman could have a BMI in the overweight range if she has an extra 10 pounds of muscle.

I find it much more useful to look at body fat percentage, but not everyone has access to this type of testing. Many of the inexpensive body fat scales work fairly well if used at the same time each day, though it is important to understand that in the morning, when you are dehydrated, the body fat percent will be slightly overestimated with these types of scales. Men should aim for a body fat percentage of 20 or below, and women should aim for a body fat percentage of 25 if they are premenopausal and 25 to 30 percent if they are perimenopausal or postmenopausal.

It is important for women to realize that female-specific body fat, such as breast tissue, will impact your fat percent goal. Women with a smaller bust size feel more comfortable with less than 25 percent body fat, while women with a larger bust size may find it challenging to get below 30 percent body fat. A nutrition or fitness professional can help you more accurately define your body fat goals.

To use BMI to set your weight-loss goals, refer to the BMI table on pages 100–101 and use the following BMI worksheet.

Doctor on Demand Worksheet:
Use BMI to Choose Your Weight Goal

BMI Categories:

Underweight = <18.5   Normal weight = 18.5–24.9

Overweight = 25–29.9   Obese = 30 or greater

Now, fill in the lines below:

Starting weight: _____   Starting BMI: _____

First Step goal weight for a BMI of 35: _____ (if BMI 40 or higher)

Second Step goal weight for a BMI of 30: _____ (if BMI 35–40)*

Final goal weight for a BMI of 18.5–24.9: _____

*If you are starting at a BMI below 35, choose a BMI goal of 30 as a first step. If you are starting at a BMI of below 30, calculate a final goal weight range only.

Those Mysterious Numbers

If you've gotten into the habit of weighing yourself frequently, you may have noticed that the numbers on the scale can change in mysterious ways. Your weight can vary from day to day—or even from hour to hour. This fluctuation is real, but it's not meaningful—and paying attention to it can really distract from reaching your longer-term goals.

I recommend weighing yourself no more than once or twice a week, especially if you are older, smaller, or have less weight to lose. That way, the number on the scale will be more of a reflection of your overall progress rather than a fluky reading that throws you off. Unexpected numbers can be frustrating and can rob you of your motivation.

If you see a surprisingly high number on the scale even though you've been doing everything right, here are some factors that might explain it:

- **You ate more salt than usual.** Excess salt holds water, and excess water adds pounds to the scale. Solutions: Drink plenty of water, watch salt intake, and weigh yourself again in a few days.

- **You haven't moved your bowels in a couple of days.** Constipation can cause excess stool to collect in your colon. Solutions: Drink plenty of water, eat high-fiber foods (but add fiber to your diet slowly, because doing so too quickly can trigger constipation), and weigh yourself again after you have moved your bowels.

- **Your hormones are haywire.** Monthly hormonal changes can leave women feeling bloated toward the end of their menstrual cycle. Solution: Wait a few days and weigh yourself when bloating reduces and the number on the scale is more realistic.

- **You travelled recently.** I find that many of my patients retain water for a few days after long-distance travel. Solution: Drink plenty of water, and wait a couple days to get on the scale.

- **You're gaining muscle.** Exercise builds lean muscle tissue, and muscle takes up less space than fat, so you will look leaner and drop inches. If you're building muscle, the numbers on the scale may not be dropping—but don't let it bother you, because more muscle translates to better health and increased daily calorie burn.

- **You're not being completely honest with yourself.** We aren't always straight with ourselves about, or fully aware of, what

Doctor on Demand Worksheet:
Use BMI to Choose Your Weight Goal

BMI takes weight and height into account. A "normal weight" BMI is under 25; however, if you have a lot of weight to lose, setting a BMI goal of 25 may be too overwhelming. Instead, consider setting a goal of lowering your BMI just a few points. Once you reach that point, you can decide whether you want to continue trying to lose weight or would rather just maintain your new BMI for a while. Remember, every pound you lose helps improve your overall health.

Use the chart below to determine your BMI. Find your height in the left column, move across the row to the right until you come to the figure closest to your current weight, then go to the top of the chart to find your BMI. For example, if you are 67 inches tall and weigh 172 pounds, your BMI is 27.

Height (inches)								Body Weight (pounds)									
58	91	96	100	105	110	115	119	124	129	134	138	143	148	153	158	162	167
59	94	99	104	109	114	119	124	128	133	138	143	148	153	158	163	168	173
60	97	102	107	112	118	123	128	133	138	143	148	153	158	163	168	174	179
61	100	106	111	116	122	127	132	137	143	148	153	158	164	169	174	180	185
62	104	109	115	120	126	131	136	142	147	153	158	164	169	175	180	186	191
63	107	113	118	124	130	135	141	146	152	158	163	169	175	180	186	191	197
64	110	116	122	128	134	140	145	151	157	163	169	174	180	186	192	197	204
BMI	19	20	21	22	23	24	25	26	27	28	29	30	31	32	33	34	35

Body Weight (pounds)

Height (inches)																	
65	114	120	126	132	138	144	150	156	162	168	174	180	186	192	198	204	210
66	118	124	130	136	142	148	155	161	167	173	179	186	192	198	204	210	216
67	121	127	134	140	146	153	159	166	172	178	185	191	198	204	211	217	223
68	125	131	138	144	151	158	164	171	177	184	190	197	203	210	216	223	230
69	128	135	142	149	155	162	169	176	182	189	196	203	209	216	223	230	236
70	132	139	146	153	160	167	174	181	188	195	202	209	216	222	229	236	243
71	136	143	150	157	165	172	179	186	193	200	208	215	222	229	236	243	250
72	140	147	154	162	169	177	184	191	199	206	213	221	228	235	242	250	258
73	144	151	159	166	174	182	189	197	204	212	219	227	235	242	250	257	265
74	148	155	163	171	179	186	194	202	210	218	225	233	241	249	256	264	272
75	152	160	168	176	184	192	200	208	216	224	232	240	248	256	264	272	279
76	156	164	172	180	189	197	205	213	221	230	238	246	254	263	271	279	287
BMI	**19**	**20**	**21**	**22**	**23**	**24**	**25**	**26**	**27**	**28**	**29**	**30**	**31**	**32**	**33**	**34**	**35**

Source: National Heart, Lung, and Blood Institute http://www.nhlbi.nih.gov/health/educational/lose_wt/BMI/bmi_tbl.htm

Help from a Pro

For people with complex dietary needs, consulting with a health-care professional who is trained in nutrition science can make sense. Talking with a dietitian, a nutritionist, or a physician nutrition specialist (like me) can provide personalized information and advice tailored specifically to your needs. Some of the people who may benefit from this include those who:

- Have chronic diseases that are affected by food choice and weight, such as high blood pressure, high cholesterol, or diabetes
- Are being treated for cancer, heart disease, kidney disease, or other conditions in which a high-quality diet may improve prognosis
- Have had trouble losing weight, or have yo-yo dieted over their lifetimes or followed multiple fad diets
- Have food allergies, intolerances, or sensitivities, or who avoid certain food groups because of personal taste, preference, or other reasons

we eat. Are you writing down everything you eat in your food journal? Are you forgetting about that tuna melt you ate for lunch or the candy bar you snuck in the afternoon because there was nothing else available? Are you eating a few more nuts or a little more olive oil than you realize? Listen, these things happen. But when they do, be honest with yourself about them. Write them down, learn from your mistakes, and move on. Don't fall into the trap of making excuses and being less than honest with yourself about your true eating habits.

Other Doctor on Demand Goal-Setting Worksheets

Once you have some idea of your goals, you can get more specific by putting some of your thoughts down in writing. Some people like doing this in a free form by writing in a journal, but I've found that many of my patients prefer using worksheets that help them really focus on the most important areas. On the following pages are three more worksheets that I use with my patients; I hope you'll find them as useful as they do.

Doctor on Demand Worksheet:
Envision Your Success

Now that you have defined a realistic goal weight and a few targets along the way, take some time to envision what success looks like: think about five things that you are most looking forward to when you reach any of your goals. Try to put some thought into these five things, and really imagine yourself at the weight that will make them achievable. Be as specific as you can to make these goals more tangible. You may want to refer back to these when you find motivation dropping or hit a rough spot in your weight-loss efforts. Some examples from my patients of what I call "envisioned success" include:

- Not wearing a baggy T-shirt to the beach again this summer.
- Fitting comfortably into an airplane seat or roller coaster.
- Keeping up with my kids at the park without being winded and embarrassed.
- Fitting into my favorite (expensive) dress (or suit) that I haven't worn in years.
- Walking into a business meeting (or job interview) feeling confident and in control because of my weight-loss success.
- Getting off my cholesterol and blood pressure medication so I don't feel so old and unhealthy.

Five things I'm most looking forward to when I reach my goal weight are:

1. _____
   _____
2. _____
   _____
3. _____
   _____
4. _____
   _____
5. _____
   _____

Doctor on Demand Worksheet:
Set Your Action Goals

Once you have your big-picture goals in mind, you can start figuring out the short-term and longer-term strategies you'll have to take in order to get to where you want to be. For this reason, it's useful to have shorter-term and longer-term "action goals" that define some of the actual steps you'll take on your weight-loss journey. On this worksheet, write down several realistic (and fun!) goals that you can start achieving today and in the weeks to come. Make sure that your goals are SMART: Specific, Measurable, Attainable, Realistic, and Timely. The following examples may help:

Shorter-Term Action Goals	Longer-Term Action Goals
Run a mile this month.	Run a 5K race by the end of the summer.
Try a new recipe for broccoli this week.	Take a class on cooking vegetables this month.
Go to the gym three times this week.	Learn to use the weight-training machines at the gym and add weight training twice a week for the next three months.
Fit into a pair of pants that did not fit last week.	Fit into a pair of pants that did not fit last month or six months ago.
Eat at least five servings of vegetables today.	Eat five servings of vegetables five out of seven days a week for the next month.

Five of my shorter-term goals are:

1. _____

   _____

2. _____

   _____

3. _____

   _____

4. _____

   _____

5. _____

   _____

Five of my longerer-term goals are:

1. _____
   _____

2. _____
   _____

3. _____
   _____

4. _____
   _____

5. _____
   _____

Doctor on Demand Worksheet: Celebrate Your Success

We're all very good at noticing our mistakes and brooding over our failures. But often we're not quite as adept at recognizing our successes. This worksheet, which I suggest you fill out at the end of each week, can help you focus on what you do well—the healthy foods you eat, the exercise you squeeze in, and the many other positive steps you take that lead you to your goals. Then, make note of some of the successes you'd like to achieve next week. Refer back to this worksheet throughout the week to remind yourself of your successes and your goals.

Date: _____ to _____

This Week's Successes

List at least one thing that you did well this week in all three categories. (*Examples:* Ate regularly, walked three times, planned weekend meals)

Nutrition:

1. _____

2. _____

3. _____

Continues ▶

Exercise:

1. _____

2. _____

3. _____

Behavior:

1. _____

2. _____

3. _____

Next Week's Goals

List at least one thing that you would like to work on in all three categories. Be specific to increase your chances of success. (Example: Eat more vegetables, increase amount of weights, stop negative thinking)

Nutrition:

1. _____

2. _____

3. _____

Exercise:

1. _____

2. _____

3. _____

Behavior:

1. _____

2. _____

3. _____

Coming Up Next

Now that you've spent some time thinking about your goals—big and small, short-term and long-term—and you've made a plan for recognizing and celebrating your successes, it's time to think about exercise. Some people love it, some people hate it, but we all know it's a fundamental part of good health. In the next chapter, you can take a fun quiz that will help you determine your own personal exercise style. Once you know what kind of exerciser you are, I'll share some strategies to make your exercise personality work for you, including how to overcome some of the challenges you will likely face given your particular fitness preferences.

CHAPTER 5

—⚭—

The Doctor on Demand Fitness Quiz: What's Your Exercise Style?

I have to admit that unlike many of my patients, I love to exercise. Unfortunately, after undergoing back surgery and two knee surgeries, I can't exercise as intensely as I used to when I was younger. Add to that equation the fact that I have two kids under the age of five, a husband, and a very busy career, and I'm left without much time to focus on fitness.

As a result, I've had to be very creative over the years in coming up with ways to stay fit and prevent those pesky pounds from creeping on or staying on after both pregnancies. My solution to this quandary is that I try to squeeze in exercise as often as possible. This includes walking errands, doing push-ups and sit-ups during commercial breaks (which often involves toddler wrestling and dog licking), and incorporating interval training to get in a super-efficient, high-intensity cardio workout (more on that to come).

On weekends I try to make exercise social and/or a family affair, going on hikes with friends, taking long walks with the kids exploring the neighborhood, or stealing away for an hour for a spin class. It's always a challenge.

I know it's hard to make fitness a priority in your life, especially if you don't enjoy it, but after reading this chapter, I hope you will be encouraged (and convinced) to incorporate exercise into your weight-loss plan.

Exercise actually has so many potential benefits that it's kind of astonishing that so few of us make the time for it. Only about half of adults in the United States get the recommended amount of cardiovascular exercise, and a mere 24 percent do as much strength training as we should. If the pharmaceutical companies invented a pill that delivered as many health benefits as exercise, people would be clamoring to take it!

109

If you don't exercise—maybe you can't stand it or you believe you are too busy to squeeze it into your schedule—it's time for that to change. (I admit, it is possible to lose weight without exercise, but you're far more likely to slim down, and stay slim, if you incorporate regular exercise—both cardio and strength training—into your daily life.) But just like your diet, there is no one-size-fits-all solution when it comes to exercise. That's why our first order of business needs to be to help you understand what kind of fitness activities best fit your style. That's where our quiz comes in. Grab a pen or pencil, and let's get moving!

The Doctor on Demand Fitness Quiz
What's Your Exercise Style?

Considering that our goal is to get you moving and make exercise a priority in your life for decades to come, let's first figure out what your preferences are. Why would I tell you that running on the treadmill every day needs to be your go-to fitness routine if that's the one thing you absolutely dread?

Use the following quiz to determine what fitness style best describes you. Then, once you've identified your style, read up on the activities that mesh best with your approach, as well as the challenges you may face. The quiz itself may even give you some new ideas for exercise, so please don't skip it.

As you do the quiz, remember that we're working together to find fitness activities that you can warm up to. If you don't like exercise, you may read the possible choices and think, "None of the above!" But in order to lose weight and keep it off, you really do have to embrace some kind of exercise. So even if you think exercise is torture, pick the answer that seems the *least* torturous to you!

1. On a Saturday morning, I think it might be fun to:

    a. Go on a bike ride with my family.

    b. Run or walk in a race.

    c. Download my favorite podcast and listen to it while putting 7,000 steps on my step counter.

    d. Take a hike in a national park I've never been to before.

    e. Put on an old movie and jump on the treadmill.

2. **If I joined a gym or a health club, I think I might most enjoy:**

    a. Taking a yoga class.

    b. Playing a new sport, such as basketball or racquetball.

    c. Doing interval workouts on the stationary cycle, treadmill, or elliptical trainer.

    d. Using the club's outdoor rock-climbing wall.

    e. Who wants to bother with a gym or club? I'd rather stay home and exercise.

3. **If I had time to exercise during my lunch break at work, I might choose to:**

    a. Go for a walk with a coworker.

    b. Swim laps with a coworker, and whoever does the most laps gets treated to lunch.

    c. Walk around the neighborhood and rack up 5,000 steps on my step counter.

    d. Take a walk in the botanical gardens near my office.

    e. Close my office door and use the stretchy exercise bands I keep in my desk drawer to strengthen my upper body.

4. **My friends would tell you I have a reputation for being the person who is:**

    a. "The planner" who organizes parties, outings, and get-togethers.

    b. "The competitor" who loves to play Scrabble, Monopoly, poker, or other games of skill.

    c. "The numbers person" who figures out how much the tip should be when we go out to restaurants.

    d. "The outdoors lover" who would rather camp than stay in a hotel.

    e. "The homebody" who likes to stay in and cook rather than go out to dinner.

5. **On a snowy day, if I had to choose an activity other than snuggling under the covers and watching the flakes fall, the activity I might consider doing is:**

    a. A sledding party.

    b. A ski race.

   c. Figuring out whether my usual neighborhood walk will add more steps on my step counter because of the snow.

   d. Wilderness hiking.

   e. Staying inside and dancing to my favorite music.

6. When I want to relax on a weekend afternoon, I would most enjoy:

   a. Having people over for a get-together at my house.

   b. Going to a friend's house to watch the football game.

   c. Playing Candy Crush Saga or other online games.

   d. Working in my garden.

   e. Lying on the couch reading a book.

7. While on vacation at a summer resort, I would enjoy:

   a. Taking a dance class with a dozen other guests.

   b. Participating in an archery competition, golf tournament, or tennis match that awards prizes to winners.

   c. Seeing how many steps I can accumulate walking around the perimeter of the resort.

   d. Going for a hike in the nearby state park.

   e. Trying out that all-in-one fitness training machine in the resort's gym.

8. Time flies when I'm:

   a. In my favorite Zumba class with a bunch of friends.

   b. Playing in a pickup basketball game.

   c. Burning 200 calories on the treadmill.

   d. Canoeing on a lake.

   e. Catching up with the latest celebrity news on TV while pumping away on a stationary cycle.

9. My favorite exercise gear is:

   a. My cell phone—I use it to invite friends to exercise with me.

   b. My skis, golf clubs, tennis racquet, and other competitive sporting equipment.

   c. My step counter or fitness tracker, and the apps that go with it.

   d. My hiking books.

   e. My television, radio, iPod, cell phone, or anything else that distracts me while I do home workouts.

10. My favorite workout locale is:

    a. The dance studio at my gym.

    b. A playing field or court.

    c. A workout room with electronic exercise equipment.

    d. Anyplace outdoors.

    e. My home.

11. If I won a cash prize that had to be spent on fitness, I would choose:

    a. A dance club membership.

    b. Coaching sessions from a professional athlete.

    c. A cardio machine with all the newest electronic bells and whistles.

    d. A cycling vacation.

    e. A home gym.

12. The phrase that best describes my ideal workout is:

    a. Fun.

    b. Challenging.

    c. Achievement-oriented.

    d. Adventurous.

    e. Convenient.

Scoring

Tally up the number of times you chose a, b, c, d, or e. Use the chart below to determine what kind of exerciser you are. Then, read all about your exercise profile after the chart, paying particular attention to the tips that will help you overcome the challenges your type of exerciser can face.

Your Answers	Your Exercise Type
Mostly a	The Socializer
Mostly b	The Competitor
Mostly c	The Data Collector
Mostly d	The Outdoor Adventurer
Mostly e	The Homebody
A mix of answers	The "Little Bit of Everything" Exerciser

The Socializer

You enjoy being with other people—life is a party, and you're always thinking up ways to spend time with friends. To inspire yourself to exercise, turn workouts into a social occasion. Think of them as an excuse to get together with friends, family, coworkers, neighbors, and even complete strangers for conversation and fun. As a social butterfly, you're likely to enjoy walking, jogging, or running in pairs or groups; taking group exercise classes; and planning activity-themed parties. Make your workouts fun social events and you'll find it much easier and enjoyable to exercise!

The Best Fitness Options for You:

- Exercise with a buddy. If you're interested in working out with a personal trainer, you can save money by sharing a trainer with a pal.

- Hire a personal trainer if you can afford it, even just for one 30-minute session each week or every couple of weeks. Many of my patients love socializing with their trainer, and the accountability to the trainer helps them stay on track.

- Take exercise classes at your local gym, health club, or community center.

- Join a sports team. Some community groups and health clubs organize team sports such as softball, basketball, and volleyball for adults. Look for a team where the focus is mainly on fun and fitness rather than serious competition.

- Sign up for group workouts, such as boot camps or dance fitness classes like Zumba and hip-hop.

- Take group lessons for sports such as tennis or golf. (And don't use a cart—walk the course!)

- Plan parties that center around seasonal activities, such as swimming and snow sports.

- Schedule activity dates instead of sitting in coffee shops, restaurants, or bars. Meet a friend for a walk rather than a meal (this is something I do regularly).

Challenges and Solutions:

- ❧ Socializers face a potential barrier that solo exercisers don't: they count on other people in order to make their workouts happen. That means an exercise session may fall through when a buddy catches a cold, has to work late, or forgets that Zumba class is on Tuesday nights. It also means you're tied to the schedule of a gym if you only do group classes, which can be a challenge if you only have 30 minutes on a Monday morning to exercise and your gym doesn't offer any classes then.

- ❧ Socializers have to be very organized, making sure to plan ahead, keep track of schedules, and remind co-exercisers about what's happening when.

- ❧ To avoid missing a workout because someone else's schedule changes, have a list of several exercise pals you can call. Or look for places such as health clubs, community centers, country clubs, or YMCAs that connect individuals looking to pair up for activities.

- ❧ If food is part of your social event, be sure to have healthy choices that won't derail the healthy eating plan that you and your friends are following.

- ❧ For those times when none of your fitness buddies are available, have a solo plan in place, such as watching TV on the treadmill or trying out a new class at the gym. Even though you enjoy socializing while getting fit, you don't want to skip workouts because nobody's around to play with.

The Competitor

You like to compete against other people and yourself. When you play games, you play to win, and you like challenging yourself to try new things, and participating in activities in which success and improvement can be measured and compared. Use this competitive spirit to fuel your workouts—you'll feel more inspired to work out when you're competing rather than just exercising.

The Best Fitness Options for You:

- ✦ Train for a race. Many communities sponsor 5K races (3.1 miles) that you can run or walk. Give yourself bonus points if you raise money for a charity, too. The Leukemia and Lymphoma Society's Team in Training programs (www.teamintraining.org) are a great way to get started and will help you get race-ready while supporting a very worthy cause.

- ✦ Join a sports team. Check with your gym, YMCA, or community education program for fun-focused softball, basketball, soccer, or volleyball teams.

- ✦ Organize a fitness challenge at work. Get everyone together for a softball league, a lunchtime walking club, or a weekend hike.

- ✦ Participate in higher-intensity exercise classes that require you to push beyond your comfort levels. Or, simply set goals for yourself to increase your performance over time, such as increasing the number of jumps you do while jumping rope for 60 seconds.

- ✦ Keep close track (in your exercise journal or utilizing an exercise app specific to your sport) of your steps, miles, minutes, speeds, and so on, so you can compete with yourself and your own records.

Challenges and Solutions:

- ✦ Team sports are great when you've got a team, but exercising all or most days of the week can be difficult if you need a whole lot of people to play with (or against) you. Be sure to have alternative workout options for days when participating in team sports is not possible. Or look for places such as health clubs, community centers, or YMCAs that have pickup games or that can accommodate singles looking to join teams.

- ✦ Participating in races or any other fitness competition takes planning, and many require preregistration. Joining a club, such as a local running club, can make it easier for you to find and take part in races.

- ✦ Competing against yourself can be motivating, as long as you don't feel unmotivated and depressed when you can't beat your best efforts. Remember that even if you don't beat your last time or record number of sit-ups, it's still commendable that you exercised and pushed yourself, so don't get down on yourself.

- If you take competition with others too seriously, you can alienate people and sabotage your fitness goals. Use competition to fuel your motivation, but if it gets too cutthroat, try to dial it back a notch or two.

- Competitive athletes who overtrain are at risk for injuries. As you work to improve your performance, be sure to train in a reasonable way that doesn't boost injury risk.

The Data Collector

You're the kind of person who likes to keep track of things. Put that data collection mindset to work with your workouts and you'll satisfy your desire to follow the numbers while exercising your body. Go ahead and keep track of everything—steps, laps, miles, minutes, hours, heartbeats, calories, grams, pounds, inches, and everything else you can possibly quantify. Have fun using all kinds of measuring gadgets, apps, and journals, and don't forget to clip on your step counter or fitness tracker before you even get out of bed in the morning.

The Best Fitness Options for You:

- Exercise on a tech-savvy treadmill, stationary bicycle, or elliptical trainer that keeps track of everything from the steps you take to the number of times your heart beats.

- Do HIIT workouts, which I'll explain in the next chapter. People who love numbers tend to enjoy these highly strategic workouts.

- Set number-based goals for daily, weekly, and monthly workouts.

- Use apps and online programs to track your progress and compete with others.

- Follow a data-centric workout plan, such as the Couch-to-5K Running Plan (www.coolrunning.com).

Challenges and Solutions:

- Being a slave to numbers can become boring over time. If you start getting tired of all that data, put your step counter or fitness app aside for a while.

- Tracking all those numbers can require you to spend a lot of time planted in a chair staring at your computer or smartphone. Try not to spend so much time crunching data that you don't have time to work out.

- Using a fitness tracker or step counter is a great way to measure your activity. But don't let an awareness of how many calories you've burned trick you into thinking you can eat extra food. I see this with my patients a lot: when they burn a lot of calories, they think they can afford to have a few treats. It's a common mistake that often leads to plateauing or weight gain.

 Clinical Pearl: *Count Your Steps*

No matter what type of exerciser you are, I strongly recommend getting a step counter (pedometer) or fitness tracker. Many of my patients are surprised by how few steps they take if they don't make an effort and are much more motivated to increase their daily step count when they can directly see the evidence of even small efforts throughout the day. A recent study showed that use of a step counter helped improve weight loss and decrease both body fat percentage and waist size. If possible, look for a step counter that measures aerobic steps (greater than or equal to 100 steps per minute) in addition to leisure steps so that you can more accurately track your daily cardio. ◇

The Outdoor Adventurer

The idea of cycling miles in a gym, swimming in an indoor pool, or "hiking" on an inclined treadmill leaves you feeling completely uninspired. You're happiest when you're outside with the sun on your back and the wind in your face. You may not warm up easily to the idea of exercise, but if it's a must-do, you'd rather do it outside. Let your love for the outdoors inspire you to get out and move.

The Best Fitness Options for You:

- Walking, jogging, hiking, or running outdoors, either on sidewalks, roads, trails, or tracks.

- Swimming in outdoor pools, lakes, or the ocean.

- Biking on roads or trails. (Bonus points for biking to work so exercise is built into your day effortlessly.)
- Tennis, golf (skip the cart), and other outdoor sports.
- Joining an outdoor adventure club.
- Winter sports, such as snowshoeing, alpine skiing, and cross-country skiing.

Challenges and Solutions:

- Be ready for every kind of weather. If you commit to outdoor exercise, you can't take the day off whenever it rains, snows, sleets, or is too hot or cold. Learn how to dress for the various kinds of weather you'll encounter, and invest in the clothing and footwear that will allow you to be out there every day.
- On days when weather keeps you indoors, have an alternative exercise plan in mind. If you can't walk outside, maybe you'll be almost as happy on the treadmill with a nature documentary playing on television.
- Some outdoor activities are more time consuming and many require extra travel time, making them limited to weekends. If this is the case with your exercise of choice, it's OK to exercise for a longer duration on weekends and less during the week, but you need to find time for one or two shorter workouts during the week that incorporate strength training, and you may need to up your calories a bit on weekends to support your longer workouts.
- Many outdoor activities are expensive—they require all kinds of gear and equipment. If you're trying a new activity, borrow gear from a friend or see if you can find it secondhand online or at a secondhand sports equipment dealer.
- Learn about how to hydrate yourself for outdoor exercise. Know how much water you need, and find smart ways to carry it with you. Remember to bring extra water on warmer, dryer days.

The Homebody

You're happiest when you're snuggled up at home watching a movie, reading a book, or checking out your friends' latest pictures on Facebook. You don't want to exercise outside, take classes with a bunch of strangers, or play a sport—you don't even feel like going to a gym or a health club. For you, it's all about convenience. If that's how you feel, then go with it! Use that homebody spirit to motivate your workouts. Forget about gyms and fitness classes—instead, set up a cozy little exercise room in your basement or spare bedroom, sign up for a subscription to Netflix, turn on the big-screen television, and sweat it out in the comfort of your own home.

The Best Fitness Options for You:

- Exercise on a new or used cardio machine.
- Lift free weights or small hand weights.
- Use a stability ball to do sit-ups, push-ups, and other strength-training exercises.
- Use stretchy exercise bands to do resistance training.
- Exercise along with a home DVD or fitness app.
- Use a Wii or other high-tech tool that combines video games with fitness.
- Jump rope.
- Dance.

Challenges and Solutions:

- People who exercise at home can become bored easily, so change things up as much as possible—use different videos, try various workouts, and keep challenging yourself to push harder.
- It's easy to postpone at-home workouts—since you can do them anytime you're home, they often sink to the bottom of your to-do list. Be sure to schedule your workouts in your datebook or electronic calendar, and treat your exercise appointments as seriously as you would any other kind of time commitment.
- Even though you prefer being alone when you exercise, you run the risk of getting bored or lonely every now and then. Consider adding occasional walks with friends, exercise classes, or other nonhome activities to your mix.
- If you exercise alone, you're less likely to notice if you're doing something wrong. Consider meeting with a personal trainer every six weeks or so, or work out with a knowledgeable friend who can spot any mistakes you're making in your form. (A trainer

or experienced buddy can also help you change up your routine to continue progressing—I recommend making changes every six to eight weeks.) I know personal trainers are expensive, but they really can be very helpful for someone who's trying to kick-start an exercise program. Even a couple of sessions with a trainer can make a huge difference—if you can possibly manage the cost, it's an investment in your health that can pay big dividends if it helps you become more active.

The "Little Bit of Everything" Exerciser

If you ended up with a range of answers in the quiz and don't fit easily into any one category, it means you're flexible, open to lots of new experiences, and likely to be successful doing a variety of fitness activities. Sometimes you'll be happy exercising with others, sometimes you prefer to be alone. You have a competitive side, but it's not your driving force. Maybe you like to keep track of your miles or your steps, but you're not obsessive. You'll exercise in different places at different times, depending on your mood— today you'd rather work out inside, and tomorrow you'll want to go outside.

This is definitely my fitness personality. I love hiking with friends and family on weekends and taking spinning and yoga classes when I have time. (My husband is an outdoor adventurer, so if we aren't outdoors being active on weekends he doesn't get enough exercise.) As for everyday workouts, when I'm on a tight schedule, I exercise at home—I have a treadmill in front of the TV, and I always record several episodes of my favorite shows to watch during workouts. I also exercise with DVDs—I have a Pilates DVD with a 20-minute workout and a DVD that works each body part for 10 minutes, so I work just one body part if I'm short on time or several if I have 30 minutes. I keep a set of five-pound hand weights by the bathtub to do arm and shoulder exercises while my son is in the bath. When I'm watching TV, I do push-ups, lunges, and tricep dips during commercial breaks.

I've always dreamed of doing a triathlon to satisfy my competitive inclinations, so maybe I'll add that to my workout goals this year.

Being a "little bit of everything" exerciser is fine. As long as you understand what motivates you, you can use this knowledge to create a plan that works for you. Focus on what you find most enjoyable, and be willing to shift gears along the way. No matter what your personality, preferences, challenges, and talents, there are fitness activities that will work for you.

Clinical Pearl: *Invest in Fitness*

No matter what kind of exerciser you are, there will be days when the easiest way to fit in exercise is with a quick home workout. If you can afford it, I highly recommend investing in some type of home exercise equipment. A treadmill (you can get a folding model if you don't have a lot of room), stationary bike (you can get a recumbent model instead of an upright if you find that more comfortable), or elliptical machine placed in front of the TV makes it easy to get 30 minutes of cardio while watching your favorite shows. A jump rope, workout video, TV exercise program, or mini-trampoline are less expensive options. Or check out Craigslist or other local listings for secondhand machines.

Coming Up Next

When you started the CleanStart Plan, I suggested that you begin walking every day. I hope you've done that, and that you're already seeing results and feeling convinced of the value of exercise in your life. If you haven't, don't worry: you can get started now. In the next chapter, I'll tell you all about why exercise helps so much with weight loss, and I'll give you some exciting ideas about how to incorporate it into your life in a fun, realistic way. I'll also give you some special "On Demand" workouts that you can customize to mesh with your schedule and your fitness level.

CHAPTER 6

—ɯɯ—

Get Moving: Exercise and Activity Strategies That Really Work

Now that you have a firm understanding of your personal exercise style, let's get specific and look at some of the ways you can add more activity into your life. If you're worried about how much time it will take, don't worry, I get it—finding time to be active for half an hour or more per day can be difficult. But believe me when I tell you that it is an investment that will pay off for the rest of your life.

Not only does exercise burn calories, but it builds muscle, helps burn fat, and delivers a host of health benefits, including these:

- ❧ Lower risk of heart disease, stroke, type 2 diabetes, metabolic syndrome, some kinds of cancer, and dementia
- ❧ Stronger bones that help decrease your risk of osteoporosis
- ❧ Better insulin response and lower overall blood sugar
- ❧ Higher HDL cholesterol and lower triglycerides
- ❧ Improved mood and lower risk of depression
- ❧ More energy during the day, and better sleep at night

If you don't exercise, or if you only exercise rarely, I hope you will take this as an opportunity to start or to start doing more. It doesn't matter how out of shape you are. It doesn't matter if you get winded after walking for five minutes. The secret is to start where you are and gradually increase your efforts. You'll find that over time, you'll become fitter, stronger, and more energetic.

123

Cardiovascular Exercise: Bump Up the Pump

Cardiovascular exercise is any activity that raises your heart rate. As you move your muscles during a cardio workout, they require extra oxygen. In order to get that oxygen to your muscles, your heart must pump harder to speed up the delivery of oxygenated blood throughout your body. Over time, as you "bump up the pump" and increase your heart rate during exercise, your heart gets stronger and more efficient. Your body also gets better at oxygen delivery to your working muscles with regular cardiovascular exercise, which is why as you become fitter, you feel much less winded.

In addition to oxygen, your muscles need extra fuel when you exercise, which comes to them in the form of sugar. During a cardio workout, your muscles take glucose (sugar) from the blood (or stored sugar from your muscles or liver), which helps lower your overall blood sugar.

The positive impact of exercise on blood sugar lasts for a while—one workout can lower your blood sugar for up to 24 hours because of better insulin sensitivity. And fitter muscles are also more sensitive to insulin—which is good for everyone, but especially for people with type 2 diabetes, prediabetes, insulin resistance, excess belly fat, or metabolic syndrome.

Beyond the benefits to your heart, oxygen delivery, and blood sugar, cardio helps with weight loss. In addition to burning calories *during* your workout, more vigorous exercise helps tune up your overall metabolism and boost calorie burn even hours *after* you finish your workout. This happens because of a process called EPOC (excess post-exercise oxygen consumption). Research shows that when you exercise intensely, your body burns more calories for up to 14 hours afterward. Talk about an amazing return on investment!

I encourage my patients to aim for *at least* 30 minutes of cardio exercise every day or most days of the week. These 30 minutes can be done all at one time or can be divided into three bouts of 10 minutes or two bouts of 15 minutes. Breaking exercise down into smaller increments does not diminish its benefits and is easier for most people to stick with. If you cannot find the time every day, at least make an effort to exercise more when you do have the time. In addition to aerobic exercise, I recommend strength training two or three times per week.

Clinical Pearl: *Schedule Exercise Appointments*

You're more likely to stick with exercise if you schedule your workouts in your weekly calendar. Sit down with your datebook or electronic calendar every week, look at the days ahead, and figure out when you'll exercise. Look for potential obstacles, and brainstorm solutions. If you are traveling, for example, book a hotel with a gym, or ask the concierge about local walking routes. I also love checking out new exercise classes or gyms when I travel, as they often have special trial packages or online deals. If you have evening plans, wake up 30 minutes earlier to squeeze in a quick morning workout, or go for a walk at lunchtime. If you take your workouts as seriously as you do all your other important commitments and appointments, you're much less likely to skip them.

Less Time, Better Workout: Use HIIT to Get Fit

Hopefully you're becoming convinced that cardiovascular exercise has some pretty impressive benefits for health and weight loss. But you may also be thinking that it can be mighty hard to fit all those workouts into your busy life. Believe me, I understand—as a working mom, I juggle a lot of responsibilities, just as you do, and often find it tough to squeeze a workout into an overscheduled day. But I also believe that exercise is so important that our lives depend on us making time for it.

One of the best strategies I've found for fitting in fitness is something called high-intensity interval training, or HIIT. As much as I love going for long walks and hikes, during the week I often don't have enough time. When I was younger and short on time, I was able to go for a short jog that burned the same amount of calories as a long walk in a much shorter period of time, but after having back surgery and two knee surgeries I can no longer jog, so HIIT helps me save an hour or two each week without burning fewer calories. I love the feeling of pushing myself harder during the HIIT Blasts that I explain below.

HIIT can save you lots of time, because it condenses a more challenging workout into a shorter amount of time—in fact, using HIIT can cut your exercise time in half, because it can burn nearly twice as many calories as lower-level cardiovascular exercise. Plus, I find that it makes the workout go by more quickly because you are paying so much attention to the interval countdowns.

Here's how HIIT works. HIIT is a type of cardiovascular exercise that alternates periods of intense activity with periods of less-intense recovery periods. During the high-intensity intervals, which I refer to as HIIT Blasts, you push your body harder and by the end of the blast, you should feel out of breath and your heart should be pounding. Then, during lower-intensity periods, you allow your body time to recover (not rest).

During a HIIT Blast, you push yourself hard enough that you can't keep it up for very long, but don't worry—you only need to maintain that intensity for a minute or less, and then you have time to recover. This allows you to condense an effective workout into a much shorter amount of time. Using HIIT Blasts, you can get more out of a 20-minute workout than someone else can in 30 to 45 minutes.

The nice part about HIIT training is that you're pushing yourself in a reasonable way that you can build up over time. When you first start your HIIT workouts, your HIIT Blasts may last for as little as 15 to 30 seconds, and your recovery periods can be as long as a few minutes. Then, as you get stronger, you'll discover that you can lengthen your HIIT Blasts and shorten your recovery periods.

Let's say you typically walk on the treadmill for 45 minutes at 3.0 miles per hour (mph). To turn your walk into a HIIT workout, you could do something like this:

- Warm-up: 3–5 minutes at 3.0 mph
- HIIT Blast: 30 seconds at 4.0 mph
- Recovery: 1–2 minutes at 3.2 mph
- Repeat HIIT Blast/recovery 7–10 more times
- Cool-down: 3–5 minutes at 3.0 mph

Then, once you feel comfortable with this HIIT workout, you can start intensifying it, either by increasing the length or speed of your HIIIT Blasts, increasing the speed of your recovery periods, or shortening the length of your recovery periods. In a few weeks, your HIIT workout may look like this:

- Warm-up: 3–5 minutes at 3.2 mph
- HIIT Blast: 1 minute at 5.0 mph (slow jog)

- Recovery: 1 minute at 3.5 mph
- Repeat HIIT Blast/recovery 7–10 more times
- Cool-down: 3–5 minutes at 3.2 mph

You can also increase intensity on a treadmill by upping the incline. This is especially useful for people with orthopedic injuries that prevent them from running (like me).

If you are using a stationary bike or elliptical machine, you can increase the resistance instead of increasing the speed. Adding incline or resistance intensity on a bike or elliptical could make your HIIT workout look like this:

- Warm-up: 3–5 minutes at 3.2 mph, no incline or minimal resistance
- HIIT Blast: 1 minute at 3.5–3.8 mph, 5% incline or level 10 resistance (1/2 of the maximum)
- Recovery: 1 minute at 3.5 mph, 1% incline or level 5 resistance
- Repeat HIIT Blast/recovery 7–10 more times
- Cool-down: 3–5 minutes at 3.2 mph, no incline or minimal resistance

As you can see, there are countless ways to design HIIT workouts. What they all have in common is the idea of alternating periods of intensity with periods of recovery.

Recovery, Not Rest

Keep in mind that the less-intense periods are called "recovery" and not "rest." You're still working and challenging yourself during the recovery periods. But you are giving your heart, lungs, and muscles a bit of a break so that they can perform at a higher level during those HIIT Blasts.

HIIT workouts don't have to be limited to cardio machines at the gym or in your home exercise room. You can create HIIT workouts for walking, jogging, or running outdoors or on a track, as well as biking, swimming, and other activities. You can even add HIIT to your neighborhood walks by adding bursts of speed that you keep track of in seconds, minutes, or driveways. Some of my patients who live in suburban settings jog for one block and then walk for one block. It doesn't really matter how you do it, as long as you push yourself and get it done. Biking on hilly terrain is also a great way to do a less structured HIIT workout—blast on the uphill, recover on the downhill and level sections.

If you are doing HIIT correctly, it should be challenging and should *not* be done daily for best results. I recommend HIIT two to three times a week and two to three days of more sustained cardio and strength training for best results.

Doing high-intensity interval training delivers some of the following health benefits:

- Increases your body's ability to use oxygen
- Burns the same amount of calories in half the time as single-level (sustained) exercise
- Builds heart strength
- Increases EPOC (calorie burn for hours after your workout compared to sustained cardio)
- Saves time and prevents boredom
- Improves blood sugar metabolism
- Boosts insulin sensitivity

Three HIIT Workouts on Demand

Here are three interval workouts you can try. Follow them as is, or vary them to fit your own exercise preferences. Always check with your doctor before starting any vigorous exercise program.

Basic Beginner Workout (for those who are just starting to exercise)
Total workout time: 21–25 minutes
In this workout, HIIT Blasts are one-fourth the length of recovery periods.

- Warm-up: 3–5 minutes at a comfortable pace
- HIIT Blast: 30 seconds of higher-intensity exercise
- Recovery: 2 minute of lower-intensity exercise
- Repeat HIIT Blast/recovery 5 more times (for a total of 6)
- Cool-down: 3–5 minutes at a comfortable pace

Intermediate Workout

Total workout time: 21 minutes
In this workout, HIIT Blasts are half the length of recovery periods.

- Warm-up: 3 minutes at a comfortable pace
- HIIT Blast: 30 seconds of higher-intensity exercise
- Recovery: 1 minute of lower-intensity exercise
- Repeat HIIT Blast/recovery 9 more times (for a total of 10)
- Cool-down: 3 minutes at a comfortable pace

Fit and Fast Advanced Interval Workout

Total workout time: 20 minutes
In this workout, HIIT Blasts are the same length as recovery periods.

- Warm-up: 2 minutes at a comfortable pace
- HIIT Blast: 1 minute of higher-intensity exercise
- Recovery: 1 minute of lower-intensity exercise
- Repeat HIIT Blast/recovery 7 more times (for a total of 8)
- Cool-down: 2 minutes at a comfortable pace

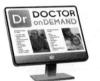

Research on Demand: Intensity Rocks Your Workout

When it comes to aerobic exercise, you can work out at one steady level of intensity (referred to as continuous exercise) or you can alternate bouts of higher- and lower-intensity exercise (referred to as interval training). Both are effective ways to boost fitness and burn calories, but research shows that interval training can provide more benefit than continuous exercise. In a 2014 study published in the *Scandinavian Journal of Medicine & Science in Sports*, researchers found that although both kinds of exercise improved blood sugar control, aerobic fitness, and some other health measures, the improvements were greater in the interval training group than in the continuous exercise group, even though both groups had burned the same amount of energy during their three-times-a-week treadmill-walking workouts.

The bottom line: To get the most from your workouts, add in some higher-intensity intervals.

Heart Rate Monitoring

One way to determine how hard to push yourself during the Blast phase of HIIT workouts—and how much to slow down during recovery—is to measure your heart rate. This isn't necessary, but if your exercise style is Data Collector, you'll probably enjoy using heart rate to guide your workouts.

To determine goal heart rates for HIIT Blasts and recovery, use the Karvonen formula below to determine your heart rate training zones (or you can use an easy online calculator).

Note: Resting heart rate is best taken in the morning at your carotid artery (at your neck) or radial artery (wrist) using your index and middle fingers. Count the beats for 30 seconds and then multiply by two.

Here's the formula to use:

HIIT Blast = [(220 – age – resting heart rate) x .8] + resting heart rate

Recovery = [(220 – age – resting heart rate) x .6] + resting heart rate

So, for example, here are the numbers for a 40-year-old with a resting heart rate of 75 beats per minute:

HIIT Blast = [(220 – 40 – 75) x .8] + 75 = 159 beats per minute

Recovery = [(220 – 40 – 75) x .6] + 75 = 138 beats per minute

Using this equation, for a 40-year-old with a resting heart rate of 75, the goal heart rate for a HIIT Blast is 159 beats per minute, and the goal for recovery is 138 beats per minute.

Don't worry if your heart rate does not drop down to the recovery zone initially. The fitter you are, the quicker your heart rate will recover. If you have heart disease or high blood pressure, consult with your doctor or an exercise professional to determine safe heart rate goals.

Fueling Your Workouts

It's important to fuel your body properly before and after you exercise. But it's also critical not to use exercise as an excuse to overeat. Here are some suggestions that can help you find the right balance:

- **Before:** If you plan to exercise intensely or for longer than 30 minutes, and it has been several hours since your last meal, try to eat a snack about 30 to 45 minutes before your workout. This will help keep your energy up as you exercise. A great option is fruit, as the carbohydrates in fruit provide energy. You can also add a little protein such as yogurt, string cheese, nut butter, or half an energy bar if you plan on working out for an hour or more.

- **After:** If you don't plan to eat for several hours after your workout, especially after a strength-training workout, I recommending consuming a high-quality protein snack like yogurt or a mini smoothie afterward to protect or build muscle and prevent excessive hunger at your next meal.

- **Extra food:** Unless you are working out really vigorously for an hour or more, there's no need to increase your daily food intake to fuel your activities. When I read the food journals of patients who are plateauing, I am not surprised to see that they are often mindlessly consuming extra calories on exercise days—for example, a 250-calorie smoothie or energy bar on top of their other daily snacks and meals. I'm also not surprised to see their weight loss kick back into gear when they recognize that their post-workout snacks must fit into their daily eating plan. Exercise snacks are not an "extra" that you earn for your virtue at the gym. The numbers just don't add up: for example, a half hour on the treadmill may burn only 100 to 200 calories, which can be wiped out with a few bites of an energy bar or a few sips of a smoothie. It is fine to snack before or after exercise, but make sure that snack is one of your daily planned snacks.

- **Empty stomach?** My patients sometimes tell me that their fitness trainers recommend they exercise first thing in the morning on an empty stomach. Is this necessary? I doubt it. I don't know of any conclusive research showing that exercising on an empty stomach has any real benefit for weight loss. Even if you burn a tiny bit more fat this way, you more than likely burn muscle too (not good), and you will probably be so hungry by the time you eat breakfast that you will consume more than you would have if you had eaten something before exercise. In addition, if your energy and blood sugar levels are lower from not eating, your workout will probably not be as vigorous and you will burn fewer calories. Try to get at least a little breakfast in before you work out, even if it is only an apple, half a protein bar, or a slice of whole-grain bread and a tablespoon of peanut butter on the way to the gym.

SOAP Notes

Runner Fuels Up with Protein and Smart Carbs

Heidi is a high school teacher, busy mom, and avid runner in her early 50s with no major medical problems who came to see me after hearing me on a radio show talking about my first book, The Busy Person's Guide to Permanent Weight Loss. *She was very frustrated that she ran up to 20 miles a week and was still 25 pounds overweight. She ate a fairly healthy diet, but it was high in carbs because she thought a high-carb diet was necessary to support her running regimen. This note is from her second visit with me, three weeks after the first appointment.*

Subjective:

Patient feels great; says my recommendation to increase protein and cut her intake of dense carbs in half is a huge change for her but her energy and her workouts are actually much better, and her cravings for sugar and carbs are much more manageable.

Objective:

Weight down 8.4 pounds. Food journal shows very good compliance with diet—dense carbs at breakfast and lunch and a few times per week at dinner. She is missing protein a few mornings a week and is not eating fruit regularly, both of which she should be doing. Eating a limited variety of foods, but overall diet is very balanced.

Assessment and Plan:

1. Exercise: Start strength training to build and maintain muscle mass for optimal metabolism and weight loss. For optimal muscle gain, eat yogurt or have a small protein smoothie after weight workout.

2. Fruit intake: Consume fruit regularly, having at least one serving per day. One option is to have fruit before her run to fuel her body, especially if she hasn't eaten in a few hours.

3. Protein at breakfast: Make sure to include protein with breakfast every day. Can add protein powder mixed with a little milk or water to her oatmeal.

Result:

Heidi lost a total of 26 pounds in 3½ months, and despite a few bumps in the road has kept the weight off for seven years.

—Melina B. Jampolis, MD

Build Lean Tissue with Strength Training

Cardiovascular exercise strengthens your heart and lungs, and it strengthens many of your muscles as well. But to build significant strength in all of your muscles, it is essential that you add strength training to your weekly exercise regimen.

Building muscle isn't about looking like a bodybuilder—although if that's what you want to do, go for it. The rest of us need to build muscle, too. We tend to think of muscles as big, bulging biceps and sculpted abdominal six-packs. But that's a limited view. If weight loss and good health are your goals, building muscle throughout your body is an incredibly helpful strategy.

When you increase the amount of muscle in your body, you also increase the number of calories your body will burn throughout the day. That's because maintaining muscle requires more energy than maintaining fat. Even when you're sitting still, your muscle cells use up more energy than your fat cells. That's why men have a faster metabolism, and often lose weight more easily, than women: they have about 30 percent more muscle.

Gaining and maintaining muscle mass is vital for both weight loss and healthy weight maintenance. If you don't work on using and building your muscles while you're losing weight, you may actually lose muscle mass, which can decrease your metabolism and make it easier to gain weight back quickly.

The best way to build muscle is through strength training, which is also referred to as resistance training. Strength training does not require a major time commitment. Once you know what you're doing, you can complete a full-body strength-training workout in just 20 to 30 minutes.

Strength-Training Tips

Even if you've never tried strength training before, you can make it part of your weekly exercise regimen. Here are a few tips to help get you started.

- **Make a plan.** Aim to do a full-body strength-training workout (20 to 30 minutes) two or three times per week. If you prefer, you can also choose one or two body parts (for a total of 5 to 10 minutes) five days per week. Ideally, try to perform one or two exercises per major body part, including back, chest, triceps (back of upper arms), biceps (front of upper arms), shoulders, legs, glutes (the cool name for your butt), and abdominals.

- **Multitask.** If you are on a tight schedule, find exercises that work two or three body parts at one time (like a lunge with a bicep curl).

- **Rep for success.** Aim for three sets of 10 to 15 repetitions (reps) per exercise, and use a weight that is challenging but not too hard to lift.

- **Speed it up.** For a faster workout—and to burn more calories— try to rest for less than 30 seconds between sets or exercises.

- **Ask an expert.** If you have never lifted weights before, consider hiring a trainer (even just once) who can teach you proper form— just a few sessions are enough to learn the basics. You can also sign up for small-group strength-training lessons at gyms, health clubs, and YMCAs.

- **Change it up.** Alternate exercises regularly to boost your progress—fitness magazines and websites are great resources for adding variety to your workouts.

Build Core Strength and Flexibility with Yoga or Pilates

Flexibility is also an important part of any fitness regimen. Though they require a bit more time, Pilates and more vigorous forms of yoga, such as Bikram and Ashtanga, can help improve flexibility and build and maintain muscle mass. Pilates is especially good for giving muscles a longer, leaner appearance and building core abdominal strength to prevent back injury. Yoga may be particularly beneficial for stress management and stretching to prevent injury and improve balance.

You may want to attend a few classes at your local gym or YMCA to learn proper form. If you don't have time for classes, there are lots of excellent instructional videos available. For the best selection, go to www.collagevideo.com. My favorite time-efficient series is the Crunch Pilates series, which offers 10 minutes per body part (chest, butt, and abs) and the Winsor Pilates 20-minute workout. The 10 Minute Solution series also fits easily into any schedule.

 ## Clinical Pearl: *Build Muscle Now, Feel Better Later*

As you age, it becomes harder to regain lost muscle due to hormonal changes, so it is best to prevent muscle loss in the first place. If you have never done any strength training, it is never too late to start. Research shows that people can build muscle well into their 70s and 80s. ◇

Get NEAT to Get Lean

So now that we're all on the same page about how important exercise is for good health and weight loss, let's talk about something else you can do that doesn't require a trip to the gym, a spin on the stationary cycle, or even a walk outdoors. You can boost your daily calorie burn by taking steps to increase your NEAT.

What is NEAT? It stands for "non-exercise activity thermogenesis," and it includes all the energy you spend doing things *other than* exercise, sleeping, and eating—for example, when you're cooking dinner, carrying laundry up the stairs, even fidgeting. Although these activities don't burn a large number of calories by themselves, they do add up over time. And people who engage in many NEAT behaviors throughout the day are more likely to succeed at losing weight and keeping it off long-term than those who don't.

When researchers looked at the number of NEAT calories that people burn, they discovered something fascinating: NEAT can vary by hundreds or even thousands of calories each day. For example, people with active jobs can burn 1,000 calories more each day than people with sedentary jobs. People who enjoy active hobbies burn more calories, too. Spending an evening watching television burns only about 30 NEAT calories, but a few hours of gardening, home repair, or other active pursuits can burn hundreds of NEAT calories.

NEAT activities can't replace exercise—although NEAT does burn calories, it doesn't strengthen your heart and lungs as cardiovascular exercises do, and it's not likely to build muscle as strength training does. But it can push up your daily calorie burn, which can make the difference between losing weight and plateauing. I had a patient when I began my career as a weight-loss doctor 14 years ago who was a meter reader for the power company, and he was on his feet the entire day walking from house to house. He was steadily losing weight on my program until he was promoted to a desk job and all of a sudden, without changing his diet, the weight loss stopped. Without all that NEAT, he had to make significant adjustments to his diet plan and he had to add in a lot more exercise to start losing again.

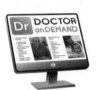

Research on Demand:
A NEAT Way to Reduce Hunger

Interspersing five-minute walks throughout your day burns calories—but it may also help you control hunger, according to a 2013 study published in the journal *Obesity*. In this study, researchers asked obese subjects to walk for five minutes 12 times per day (for a total of 60 minutes) and measured their hunger levels throughout the day. On other days, the subjects walked 60 minutes all at once or they did no walking at all. The researchers found that on days when study subjects took multiple five-minute walks, they reported feeling less hungry than the other days. And both kinds of exercise appeared to help them feel more satiated than doing no exercise at all.

The bottom line: Although exercise burns calories, being active throughout the day probably won't make you hungrier than sitting around doing nothing—in fact, it may even reduce hunger.

NEAT Ways to Get Fit

How can you make NEAT work for you? Here are some suggestions:

- ❧ **Leave the car at home.** When going to work, running errands, and visiting friends, try to choose a form of transportation that gets you moving. If you take a train or bus to work, try walking to the station or stop instead of driving. When possible, get off one stop early and walk the rest of the way. In parking lots, go for the spots farthest from your destination rather than right up close. (We all know how great it feels to luck out and get that right-up-front parking space. But when you're looking for NEAT ways to get fit, you drive right by that space and head for one at the other end of the lot.)

- ❧ **Socialize on the move.** Rather than meeting a friend for a sedentary cup of coffee at your local java shop or a glass of wine at a restaurant, go for a talk-walk and burn calories while you catch up. Or, plan an activity that has you on your feet rather than in a seat: meet for a game of pool or darts, visit an exhibit at a local museum, or go window-shopping.

- ❧ **Seek out stairs.** Skip the escalators and elevators, and burn some calories walking up the stairs instead.

- ❧ **Pace instead of standing.** When you're waiting for a bus, stuck in line at the grocery store, or stranded in the waiting room of a doctor who's running late, pace or walk around instead of sitting. If you have to stay in one spot, shift your weight from foot to foot or march in place. (Nothing drives me crazier than seeing everyone sitting at the airport waiting to sit on a plane for hours! Walk around, window-shop, or just stand up and watch the planes take off and land!)

- ❧ **Stand instead of sitting.** Pay attention to the times of day when you sit a lot, and try standing or walking during those times. For example, walk around while talking on the phone. If you spend your workday sitting at a desk, consider a standing desk or a treadmill desk—or simply stand rather than sitting while you read reports or speak with colleagues.

- **Take frequent breaks from sitting.** Set a timer on your phone or computer, and get up and walk around every 30 to 60 minutes. You can go to the bathroom, fill up your water bottle, or even do some simple stretches that will activate your body and your mind.

- **Turn off the TV.** Curling up on the couch and watching your favorite show or movie can be relaxing, and it's fine to do occasionally. But if you're spending hours sitting in front of the TV every day, look for some other, more active ways to spend your time: walking the dog, playing with your children, gardening, going dancing, and doing yard work, to name a few. When watching TV, get up during each commercial break and walk around or do some stretches.

- **Carry things.** Lifting weights at the gym is just one way to build muscle. Whenever you have the chance, do your "lifting" out in the world—for example, carry groceries in a basket rather than wheeling around a cart.

- **Choose active volunteer work.** Volunteer to walk dogs at your local shelter, stock shelves at the hospital gift shop, or get involved with kids at your church's Sunday school.

- **Do active chores.** Wash your car by hand, mow the lawn, paint, wash windows—sure, it's easier to have other people do these jobs for you, but doing them yourself can burn calories and save money.

- **Get your family moving, too.** Switch to family bowling night instead of family movie night, or go for miniature golf instead of a matinee.

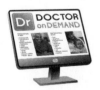 ## Research on Demand: Stand Up for Health

The simple act of sitting appears to have a negative impact on health. The longer we sit, the more likely we are to develop chronic illnesses such as diabetes and heart disease. Sitting even contributes to the aging of our cells, according to a 2014 study published in the *British Journal of Sports Medicine*. That study found that sitting time contributed to cellular aging—people who sat longer had shorter telomeres, which are the structures found at the ends of chromosomes. Shorter telomere length is believed to be associated with shorter life span.

The bottom line: Whenever possible, choose standing or walking over sitting.

Put It in Writing

Just as I recommend that my patients write down what food they eat in a food journal, I also recommend recording exercise in a fitness journal. This allows you to honestly see how much exercise you do. Just as we tend to *underestimate* the amount of food we eat, we tend to *overestimate* the amount of exercise we do. Writing it down helps to keep you honest. Keeping track of your workouts reinforces your accomplishments and helps you identify areas where you can improve.

Recording your activities can be a real motivational force as well. Tracking your progress over time—either in minutes, miles, or steps— can show you how far you've come and how much you've accomplished. I encourage you to set daily, weekly, and monthly goals, and to use your exercise journal to see how close you're coming to meet these goals.

Many people like to include exercise info in their food journal; others prefer to track food and exercise separately. Either is fine, and it's up to you to choose what you prefer. Keep them both close at hand so you can fill them out throughout the day. Use a notebook, a journal, your phone, or an app—whatever works best for you.

On the next two pages you'll find a weekly exercise journal with sample entries, along with a blank journal page you can copy and use.

Weekly Exercise Journal—Sample Entries

Day	Activity	Time Total
Sunday	Morning: Went for a 45-minute walk to the coffee shop and back with Linda. After dinner, rode stationary bicycle for 15 minutes while watching TV. Bedtime: Walked dog for 10 minutes.	Cardio total: 70 mins
Monday	Lunchtime: Went to gym; did 20-minute HIIT workout on treadmill, followed by strength-training routine. Bedtime: Walked dog for 10 minutes.	Cardio total: 30 mins Strength total: 20 mins
Tuesday	Morning: Took a brisk 20-minute walk before work. Bedtime: Walked dog for 10 minutes.	Cardio total: 30 mins
Wednesday	Tired today, no exercise	Cardio total: 0 mins
Thursday	Morning: Walked dog for 20 minutes. Lunchtime: Went to gym; swam laps for 20 minutes, followed by strength-training routine. Bedtime: Walked dog for 10 minutes	Cardio total: 50 mins Strength total: 20 mins
Friday	Lunchtime: Jogged/walked on treadmill for 30 minutes. Early evening: Took dog to park and walked for 30 minutes.	Cardio total: 60 mins
Saturday	Afternoon: Went for a 50-minute bike ride by the river with Becky. Bedtime: Walked dog for 10 minutes.	Cardio total: 60 mins
	Cardio total for week	**300 mins**
	Strength total for week	**40 mins**

Weekly Exercise Journal

Day	Activity	Time Total
Sunday		
Monday		
Tuesday		
Wednesday		
Thursday		
Friday		
Saturday		
	Cardio total for week	
	Strength total for week	

Coming Up Next

Meeting your weight-loss goals isn't just about eating right and exercising, although of course those matter a huge amount. The truth is, your mind plays as big a part in weight loss as your body, and if your mind isn't in the right place, it's much harder for you to slim down your body. In the next chapter, we'll look at some of the psychological and emotional challenges that can stand in the way of weight loss, and I'll give you a slew of behavior changes you can make to get yourself on the right track.

CHAPTER 7

—ᄤ—

Get Your Head in the Game: Understanding the Psychological Side of Weight Loss

One of the most important lessons I've learned from my patients is that weight loss is much easier when you have your head in the right place. We think of weight loss as being all about food and exercise—and those things are critically important, of course—but the truth is that your mindset can have as much impact on your weight as the food you eat and the physical activities you do. By creating emotional, social, and physical environments that support your efforts to change your diet and rev up your activities, you'll increase your chances of success.

I am not a trained psychologist, but working in the field of weight loss for the past 14 years has given me a deep understanding of the importance of the psychological/behavioral aspect of weight loss.

Since thoughts can matter as much as food and fitness, this chapter is about identifying and restructuring the thinking patterns, emotional issues, and behaviors that may stand in the way of successful weight loss. In two steps, we'll work together to put you in the best possible state of mind to meet your weight-loss goals.

We'll start by taking a good look at what's going on with your thoughts and habits regarding food, eating, and weight loss. Once we have an understanding of your weight-loss mind-frame, I'll recommend strategies that can help get you into a better place.

Some of these strategies involve reaching out to others. For example, if it seems you are engaging in disordered eating, I'll advise you to seek help from a health-care professional—either from your own provider, or with the help of a Doctor on Demand psychologist. But most of the suggestions in this chapter are simple changes in thinking habits and behavior patterns that can pay off big time as you tackle your weight-loss goals.

STEP 1: *Know Your Mind*

Most diets work to some extent for most people, but staying on them and maintaining healthy eating and exercise habits for a lifetime usually involves the brain more than the stomach.

When I evaluate new patients, I spend at least an hour with them asking about their dieting history and personal eating challenges. I also evaluate them for possible psychological issues that can easily get in the way of successful weight loss.

Since I can't see you as a patient, I have put together a few quizzes to help you figure out if you may be dealing with conditions that require more attention and perhaps even professional help. While these quizzes are not meant to provide a medical diagnosis, I think they can be useful tools to help you figure out the best comprehensive weight-loss strategy for you.

We can test the strength of the human body by seeing how much weight we can lift or how fast we can run. But measuring mental health can be a bit more difficult. Health-care professionals can't use a blood test or an X-ray to diagnose a mental health disorder; instead, they use information provided by the patient as well as their powers of observation, along with various screening tools and questionnaires to determine the presence of disordered thinking.

Among people who are overweight or obese, I find that three psychological disorders occur most commonly: binge eating disorder, food addiction, and depression. People who have these disorders struggle much more with weight loss than people who don't have them. That's why it's important to determine whether they are an issue for you. Let's start with binge eating, which is fairly common among overweight and obese people.

Binge Eating: When Overeating Veers Out of Control

Binge eating is a situation in which someone eats a lot of food in a short amount of time. Picture someone who buys a dozen cupcakes, climbs into her bed, and eats every single one—that's what binge eating looks like.

Specific definitions vary, but in general binge eating occurs when a lack of control leads to the consumption of a very large amount of food within a two-hour period. Binge eating is more extreme than overeating; someone who engages in binge eating may consume a day's worth of calories or more in just an hour or two.

Many of the patients I've seen over the years have binge eating tendencies. (Having a *tendency* to binge eat, rather than a binge eating *disorder*, means people do it sometimes, but not to the serious degree that would fit the criteria of a diagnosis of binge eating disorder.) However, even among people who have the tendency and not the disorder, binge eating can still be very problematic when it comes to weight loss, and it needs to be addressed.

Binge eating disorder affects up to 4 percent of the general population, but it is more prevalent among people who are overweight or obese. It is associated with higher levels of anxiety and depression.

Binge Eating: Questions to Ask

We all overeat sometimes. But when overeating occurs frequently and is accompanied by shame and guilt, it may be a sign of binge eating. Only a health-care professional can determine whether you have binge eating disorder. However, answering the following questions can help you get a sense of whether binge eating may be a problem for you.

- ⤞ Do you engage in binge eating twice a week or more?
- ⤞ Have you experienced binge eating episodes for at least three months?
- ⤞ Do you have eating experiences in which you eat much more quickly than normal?
- ⤞ Do you sometimes eat until you feel uncomfortably full?
- ⤞ Do you sometimes eat large amounts of food even though you don't feel physically hungry?
- ⤞ Do you eat alone sometimes because you are embarrassed to have others see how much you eat?
- ⤞ After overeating, do you sometimes feel disgusted with yourself, depressed, ashamed, or guilty?

Your Answers

If you answer yes to several of these questions, especially if you answered yes to the first two questions—or if you think you have a serious problem with binge eating—I strongly suggest you speak with a health-care professional, either in person or through Doctor on Demand. With the help of a psychologist or other medical care provider who has experience treating eating disorders, people with binge eating disorder can learn to understand and change their behavior. They may also be treated with medication.

If you answer yes to one or two of these questions, you can probably improve your overeating tendencies by following the suggestions in Step 2.

Research on Demand: Think Before You Eat

The way you think about food can have an impact on how you eat, according to a study released at the Obesity Society's 2014 annual meeting. Researchers used functional magnetic resonance imaging (fMRI) scans to watch the brains of overweight or obese study participants as they viewed photos of enticing foods such as French fries, pizza, and ice cream. They found that by thinking about the long-term negative impact of eating these foods, subjects were able to increase activity in the parts of their brains that are involved in inhibition and self-regulation. Similar studies have found that these kinds of thinking strategies help people quit smoking.

The bottom line: Before you eat something you're trying to avoid, spend a few moments thinking about its potential long-term negative impact on you. Sure, the ice cream cone will be delicious, but how will you feel about it later, when you're writing it down in your food journal? How will you feel about it next week, when your favorite pants don't fit so well? Really try to picture it.

Food Addiction: An Uncontrollable Desire

Just as we can develop addictions to alcohol, drugs, tobacco, gambling, and sex, evolving research suggests that we have the potential to develop an addiction to food. Although food addiction is often less obvious than other eating disorders, it is an issue for many people. If you're one of them, the first step toward helping yourself is identifying your problem and asking for help.

Get Help with Eating Disorders

The National Eating Disorders Association (NEDA) is the leading nonprofit organization in the United States that advocates for and supports people and families affected by eating disorders. NEDA provides education, screening guidelines, information about support groups, treatment and recovery resources, and a toll-free helpline (800-931-2237). To find out more, visit NEDA's website: www.nationaleatingdisorders.org.

Food addiction is a somewhat controversial condition that has not been thoroughly studied—in fact, a formal psychological diagnosis for food addiction has not been established. What we do know, though, is that it is becoming more and more apparent that certain foods, especially sweet foods and highly palatable foods that are high in sugar, fat, and salt, have a more powerful effect on brain chemistry in many people, particularly those who are overweight or obese, than they do on others. Some people describe that effect as an addiction—many of my patients tell me that they feel like they are "addicted" to sugar or other types of foods that are high in fat and salt. They tell me that they just can't seem to give them up and often need larger amounts to feel satisfied.

While the differences can be subtle, this is different from the patients who tell me that, on occasion, they are completely consumed by thoughts of wanting their favorite frozen yogurt, and then go 30 blocks out of their way to get it as an occasional treat because they really enjoy that particular yogurt. In this case, they are making a conscious and controlled choice to treat themselves, without the guilt. If they were addicted to frozen yogurt, the sight of any frozen yogurt shop would lead to an immediate desire to enter the store, even if they were running late for a meeting and had just consumed a big lunch. They would probably eat a large serving even if it didn't taste that great, and would feel remorseful afterward.

I must admit, every time I'm in New York, I fantasize about and always make time for a visit to my favorite chocolate chip cookie shop in the world. When I arrive, I savor the cookie, which definitely tastes addictive, but then I go home, maybe even with an extra cookie or two that I freeze for a special occasion, and do an extra hour or two of exercise the next week and often forget about the cookies in the freezer for months.

However, for people who experience an addiction to food, eating certain types of foods elicits a response similar to that of other addictive substances such as drugs, alcohol, and nicotine. One of these responses is the inability to control consumption even when we *know* that the substance is not healthy. People who are addicted to food may feel cravings for that food even when they are full, eat more of their problem foods than they had intended, and feel guilty or shameful when they eat them.

People who are addicted to drugs or alcohol can learn to avoid them completely, but because we have to eat to live, people who are addicted to food have to take a more nuanced approach to controlling their addiction. They can't stop eating, but they can learn to avoid the foods and situations that trigger their addictive behavior.

To help you figure out whether food addiction may be an issue for you, I've included a list of questions you can ask yourself about your eating behavior. There is considerable overlap between binge eating and food addiction, so if you feel that you are a binge eater, it is especially important to consider the role of food addiction. If the answers to these questions lead you to believe that food addiction may be a concern, you can see a health-care professional or use the suggestions in Step 2 to help reverse some of the eating habits that lead you to consume problem foods.

Most Addictive Foods

According to Yale University researchers, the foods most likely to elicit feelings of addiction include:

- ✦ Sweets such as ice cream, candy, chocolate, cookies, donuts, and cake
- ✦ Starches such as white bread, bagels, rolls, rice, and pasta
- ✦ Salty snacks such as pretzels, chips, and crackers
- ✦ Fatty foods such as steak, burgers, bacon, French fries, and pizza
- ✦ Sugary drinks such as sweetened soda

The questions below are based on the Yale Food Addiction Scale, a questionnaire developed by researchers at the Rudd Center for Food Policy and Obesity. The full questionnaire and information on scoring is available at http://www.yaleruddcenter.org/what_we_do.aspx?id=263.

Food Addiction: Questions to Ask

- When you eat certain kinds of foods, do you find that you eat more than you had planned, have trouble stopping, and sometimes eat so much that you feel sick?
- Have you frequently tried and failed to avoid eating certain foods?
- Do you frequently think about certain kinds of food and go out of your way to obtain them?
- Do you become so consumed with thoughts about either eating certain foods or avoiding them that it has a negative effect on your work, family life, or social life?
- Do you find that you have to eat more and more of certain foods in order to feel satisfied by the foods?
- Do you hide your consumption of certain foods from friends, family, coworkers, and other people?
- Do you experience withdrawal-like symptoms such as anxiety or agitation when you stop eating the foods you're most drawn to?
- Are you upset or worried about your dependence on certain kinds of food?

Your Answers

If you answer yes to several of these questions—or if you think you may have a serious problem with food addiction—I strongly suggest you speak with a health-care professional. With the help of a psychologist or other medical care provider with experience treating eating disorders, people with food addiction can learn to understand and change their behavior. They may also be treated with medication.

If food addiction is not a problem for you but you do occasionally find yourself going overboard with certain kinds of food, you can work to improve your overeating tendencies by following the suggestions in Step 2.

The Story Behind Food Addiction

Former US surgeon general Dr. David A. Kessler wrote an outstanding book on the topic of food addiction titled *The End of Overeating: Taking Control of the Insatiable American Appetite*. In it, he explains how food addiction has developed, and he describes the essential behavioral components for reversing habits. I recommend it for anyone who wants to learn more about this problem, either from a personal standpoint or for its implications for public health.

Research on Demand: Food Addiction by Numbers

How prevalent is food addiction? Researchers at Yale University wanted to find out, so they administered their questionnaire, the Yale Food Addiction Scale, to 134,175 women enrolled in the long-running Nurses' Health Study. The researchers found that overall, 5.8 percent of the women met the criteria for food addiction.

The bottom line: Food addiction is more common than you may realize, especially among people who are overweight or obese. If you think you may be displaying food-addictive behaviors, talk to a health-care professional.

Depression: More Than Just the Blues

Everyone feels sad sometimes—that's completely normal and part of being human. But when feelings of sadness don't go away, or when they interfere with daily life, they may be a sign of depression.

Depression is an illness that strikes millions of Americans. We don't know exactly what causes depression, but we do know that certain factors—including genetics, a history of abuse, elevated levels of life stress, substance abuse, and hormonal changes—are associated with higher depression rates.

Weight appears to play a part for some people as well. Studies have found higher rates of depression among people who are obese, although researchers don't know for sure if being overweight makes people depressed, or if depressed people overeat as a way of self-medicating. I believe it's a little of both.

I see a lot of depression in the patients in my practice. Although the cause-and-effect relationship between weight and depression is not entirely clear, addressing depression can help with weight loss. If you are depressed, you may need treatment.

Depression is nothing to be ashamed of or to feel guilty about—it's a health condition, not a character flaw. People don't become depressed because they are weak, lack self-discipline, or don't try hard enough to feel good; depression is an illness, and if you have it, treatment can help you feel better.

As with other mental health conditions, you can't self-diagnose depression—only a health-care professional can do that. But, using the screening tool below can help give you a feel for whether depression is a concern for you.

Patient Health Questionnaire for Depression

During the past two weeks, how often have you been bothered by any of the following problems?

	Not at all	Several days	More than half the days	Nearly every day
1. Little interest or pleasure in doing things.	0	1	2	3
2. Feeling down, depressed, or hopeless.				
3. Trouble falling asleep or staying asleep, or sleeping too much.				
4. Feeling tired or having little energy.				
5. Poor appetite or overeating.				
6. Feeling bad about yourself—or that you are a failure or have let yourself or your family down.				

Continues ▶

	Not at all	Several days	More than half the days	Nearly every day
7. Trouble concentrating on things, such as reading the newspaper or watching television.				
8. Moving or speaking so slowly that other people could have noticed. Or the opposite—being so fidgety or restless that you have been moving around a lot more than usual.				
9. Thoughts that you would be better off dead or hurting yourself in some way.				

Total Score: [ ]

About Your Score

Only a health-care professional can diagnose depression. If your score on this questionnaire is 10 or higher, or if you circled answer 1, 2, or 3 on question 9, I recommend that you schedule an appointment with your primary care doctor or other health-care provider to be screened for depression. If you receive a diagnosis of depression, your doctor may prescribe medication and/or therapy.

If do not have depression but occasionally feel blue, here are some strategies that can help you as you work on losing weight:

- ✦ **Get up and move.** Exercise has the power to boost mood—in fact, it's often referred to as a natural antidepressant. When you feel blue, it can be difficult to motivate yourself to move, but it's well worth it: even just a few minutes of walking, swimming, jogging, or other aerobic exercise can help you begin to feel better. Start with something simple, such as a five-minute walk. Chances are that once you get moving, you'll want to keep going.

- **Rely on social support.** Spending time with loving family and supportive friends can be just what you need when you feel down. On the other hand, social isolation can exacerbate negative feelings.

- **Get enough sleep.** Being tired has a huge impact on your mood, so do your best to get the rest you need. Most adults need seven to eight hours of sleep per night, but many of us scrimp by on much less. If you have trouble falling asleep, staying asleep, or waking up too early, or if you get enough rest but still feel tired all the time, discuss it with your doctor, because you may have a sleep disorder that can be improved with treatment.

- **Try mind/body strategies for stress relief.** Meditation, visualization, mindfulness, and other mind/body techniques can help elicit the relaxation response, a release of brain chemicals and physiological changes that reduce feelings of stress.

- **Up your omega-3s.** Some research suggests that omega 3 fatty acids play a role in prevention and treatment of mild to moderate depression, so I recommend that you seek them out. The best sources are fatty fish such as salmon, herring, anchovies, mackerel, and tuna. If you don't like fish, talk with your doctor about supplementing your diet with fish oil capsules. Omega-3 can also help fight inflammation, which could decrease the negative health impact of depression.

- **Get your Bs.** Deficiencies in B vitamins, including B6, B12, and folate (also known as folic acid), have been associated with higher levels of depression, so make sure you're eating a diet rich in these vitamins, or take a daily multivitamin with at least 50 percent of the recommended daily allowance (RDA) of these mood-friendly nutrients. RDA and top food sources for each can be found in the box on the next page.

The Place to Be for B Vitamins

Looking for B vitamins? Here's the RDA and top food sources of these important nutrients:

Vitamin B12

- RDA 2.4 micrograms/day for males and females ages 14 and older
- Good food sources: meat, poultry, seafood, low-fat dairy, fortified cereals

Vitamin B6

- RDA 1.3 milligrams/day for males and females age 19–50
- Good food sources: avocados, sweet potatoes, peanut butter, sesame seeds, cabbage

Folate

- RDA 400 micrograms/day for males and females ages 14 and older
- Good food sources: spinach, asparagus, peanuts, sunflower seeds, chickpeas

How Is Depression Treated?

For my patients with mild depression, I typically recommend nondrug approaches. I start with lifestyle strategies such as diet adjustments and exercise. I sometimes recommend over-the-counter supplements such as St. John's wort. Studies have found that St. John's wort can help with some kinds of depression, although the evidence is not definitive. One study found that it may be helpful in treating perimenopausal and postmenopausal depression. Keep in mind that even though St. John's wort is "natural," it can interact with prescription medications, so be sure to talk with a doctor if you are considering trying it.

When people have moderate or severe depression, medication and/or therapy can help. (Make sure you don't combine St. John's wort with prescription antidepressants, because it can cause potentially life-threatening side effects.) If you feel depressed, or if you believe depression is interfering with your ability to get to a healthy weight, talk to your primary care doctor

Clinical Pearl: *When You're Feeling Depressed,*
Don't Scrimp on Dense Carbs

I know I suggested cutting back on or cutting out dense carbs when you're trying to speed up your weight loss. But if you're feeling depressed, you may want to hold on to your dense carbs on cycling days. Eating healthy amounts of dense carbs, such as whole grains, beans, and starchy vegetables—as well as fruit and non-starchy veggies—may have a positive effect on mood, so don't cut them out completely. But don't use this as an excuse to eat sugar and refined grains: not only can it lead to inflammation and insulin resistance, eating these unhealthy foods has also been associated with depression. ◇

for a referral to a therapist, psychologist, or psychiatrist. Or, consider using the Doctor on Demand app for psychological help in the comfort of your own home.

Some people who take antidepressant medication seem to gain weight as a side effect of the medication. This is a very unwelcome situation, especially for people who hoped that treating their depression would help them lose weight rather than gain it. If weight gain occurs after starting an antidepressant, talk with your doctor. When appropriate, your doctor may consider switching to a different medication—some are less likely than others to cause weight gain.

STEP 2: *Use Smart Strategies to Curb Overeating, Binge Eating, and Food Addiction*

Whether you have just the occasional tendency to overeat or you are working with a health-care professional to deal with binge eating or food addiction, here are some strategies that can help you take charge of your eating. Many of these are based on the addiction research discussed in much greater detail in Dr. David Kessler's book *The End of Overeating*.

Know your triggers. Using your food journal or worksheet, identify any foods that may trigger overeating. Triggers can be sensory (the sight or smell of food) or situations that are discussed in the next point. Trigger foods vary, but some common ones are potato chips or other salty snacks, ice cream, candy, French fries, cookies, fast food, nuts, or the smell of pizza, fresh-baked cookies, or cinnamon rolls.

Once you identify your trigger foods, consider eliminating them from your house or limiting your exposure (taste, sight, and smell) as much as possible. If your family won't let you get rid of all the temptation, make sure to place it out of sight as much as possible in your pantry or freezer—but be sure to explain to them how important it is for you to remove the foods, and ask them for their support. Research shows that when tempting foods are not visible or not in close proximity, people consume far less of them. You're less likely to be tempted or to binge if doing so requires you to drive to a store.

 Clinical Pearl: *Control the Remote*

If you are prone to overeating or binging, I recommend fast-forwarding through commercials for your trigger foods. Studies show that the brains of overweight people respond differently to pictures of tasty treats than do the brains of slim folks. When it comes to trigger foods, if you can't control portions or have just one bite, it is better to avoid even seeing images of them until healthier eating behavior habits are in place. The same goes for your computer: control your clicks by avoiding popular websites devoted to tempting food imagery.

Identify "at-risk" situations. Using your food journal or worksheet, determine if certain situations predispose you to bingeing or overeating. For example, you may be more likely to overeat when you are tired, stressed, blue, lonely, working late, watching TV, drinking alcohol, feeling like you need a reward, or doing something you don't enjoy. High-risk situations can also include daily habits like your morning visit to the café that usually involves a pastry, heading straight to the fridge when you get home from the office, or even an eating memory like Sunday dinner with the family that always ends with a slice of pie.

Once you know what your high-risk situations are, you can either try to limit or avoid them or work on developing a plan of action to overcome them.

Plan for success. Experts believe that you only have a brief window of time to decide not to give in to tempting situations, so as often as possible decide quickly and firmly not to give in. Also, try to preplan how you will handle high-risk situations. If Friday dinner at your friend's always involves tempting dessert, offer to bring a healthier dessert instead or resolve to skip the sweet treats and have a cup of chamomile tea instead.

Learning new behaviors may be challenging at first, but with practice they will become easier over time. If you always head straight to the pantry when you get home from work, develop a new pattern such as opening the mail or, better yet, throwing on your workout clothes and doing a little exercise. Sometimes, just getting busy with a chore or activity can help take your mind off overeating: vacuuming, walking the dog, polishing your nails, washing your car—anything that redirects your focus away from food.

Stop and think. If you find yourself tempted to binge, try to take a minute to think about the negative consequences of your choice and reinforce the value, both short-term and long-term, of not overeating. Tell yourself that you CAN successfully resist.

Be mindful. If you do choose to overeat or eat less healthful foods, take steps to be more mindful about your behavior. Force yourself to eat only at the dining room or kitchen table. Turn off the TV, and eat as mindfully as possible—if you allow yourself to eat while watching TV, you are making it much easier to detach yourself from your eating and much more difficult to stop eating before the major damage is done. Finally, avoid eating directly out of containers. By transferring foods to bowls or plates, you maintain some amount of portion control, which can prevent the mindless overeating that bingeing often involves.

Question yourself. After overeating or bingeing, take some time afterward to ask yourself about it and make notes on it in your food journal. What do you think triggered your overeating? How did it make you feel? What can you learn from it?

It is helpful to write down the answers to these questions because you can use the information you gather to learn about your own personal overeating patterns. You can also look back at your notes the next time you feel vulnerable—reading about your last bingeing episode might help prevent your next one.

Are Your Genes Out to Get You?

Genetics plays a considerable role in obesity, but this does not mean that you are destined to be overweight if one (or both) of your parents has a weight problem. It does mean that you are probably more susceptible to environmental factors, such as increased food availability, larger portions, and less healthy food choices, which lead to weight gain.

If being overweight or obese runs in your family, you may feel hungrier more frequently than someone who does not struggle with weight. Or perhaps you don't feel full as easily, so you eat slightly more when you are served the same amount of food as a thinner person. Your metabolism may be a bit more sluggish than other people's, or your body may not handle carbohydrates as efficiently as it could, causing you to more easily store excess carbs as fat. No, you're not imagining this—you can assume that genetics is partly to blame.

The bottom line, though, is that whatever role genetics plays, you still have some control. You may have to eat a little less or a little differently and exercise a little bit more, but permanent weight loss is possible for the great majority of overweight people. I am not saying that you can have the figure of a supermodel or pro athlete if you work hard enough, but you can have a strong, fit, healthy body—if you are committed to making changes in how you eat and live.

Make it social. Social support can be very helpful in overcoming overeating. A trusted friend or family member can help you recognize and avoid temptation, stay motivated, and even provide accountability. They may even be able to help you identify food triggers.

Try designating a close friend as a "binge buddy" whom you can call when you are tempted. Family and friends can also distract you from food. If you eat when you're home alone on Friday nights, for example, planning a Friday movie night with family members may keep you from overeating.

Close your eyes and visualize. When you're tempted to overeat, shut your eyes and try to visualize exactly how you would look and feel afterward. It can also be helpful to build a negative association with foods that are especially tempting (coffee shop muffin = muffin top). Then, visualize how you would look and feel if you were to succeed at avoiding a binge and, by doing so, moving one step closer to your weight-loss goals. Just as professional athletes mentally rehearse their performances, you can mentally rehearse avoiding a binge and walking away from food.

Forgive yourself and move forward. After overeating, it is essential that you forgive yourself and focus on getting back on track. Do not torture yourself by getting on the scale the next morning or trying on the pants that fit you perfectly two days ago. This will only bum you out, making you more susceptible to bingeing again. Remember, mistakes are normal, and you can overcome them. You have the power to turn this behavior around.

Strategy for Success: Ditch the "All-or-Nothing" Mentality

If you've ever given up your diet for the entire day (or week!) because you ate one cookie after lunch, you know exactly what the "all-or-nothing" mentality is. All-or-nothing thinking is an exaggerated thought pattern that pushes you to see things as either black or white, success or failure. It leaves no room for in-between thinking that allows for shades of grey or partial success. With an all-or-nothing attitude, if you eat a bag of chips at 1:00 p.m., you ruined your diet plan for the day, so you might as well give up, eat what you want for the rest of the afternoon and evening, and just start over tomorrow morning.

All-or-nothing thinking can really interfere with your ability to reach your weight-loss goals—or any life goals, for that matter. I have seen so many people fail at weight loss or fall short of their goals because of this deeply ingrained mentality. They expect themselves to follow every recommendation 100 percent perfectly, and if they don't, they give up.

If you engage in all-or-nothing thinking, try to become aware of it. Once you identify your all-or-nothing moments, work to try to talk yourself out of feeling that way. Remind yourself that you don't have to be perfect. As you read this book, remember that the suggestions I am making are *recommendations*, not rules set in stone. Some of them will work well for you; some won't. There will be days when you can follow them closely, and days when you can't. That's OK. Try your best, but give yourself permission to make a few less-than-perfect choices occasionally, and for goodness' sake, don't beat yourself up about it. Just try to make the best choices you can the majority of the time.

Celebrate your achievements and forgive yourself for your mistakes. When you slip up, get back on track as soon as possible. Don't blow an entire day simply because you didn't have time for an afternoon snack, got to the restaurant famished, and ate a slice or two of bread. Just try to make even better choices the rest of the meal or the next day.

If you expect yourself to be perfect, you will fail, guaranteed. No one is perfect all the time. I skip my workouts when I get overcommitted. I *love* chocolate chip cookies and pizza, and I indulge on occasion. The key is to do the best you can and to be consistent.

All-or-nothing thinking can sabotage your exercise goals, too. Be aware of it, and try to stop it in its tracks. Don't skip your workout because you only have 20 minutes instead of the hour that you had planned. If you don't have time to exercise or get to the gym habitually, do what you can to move your body and get your heart rate up at home, any chance that you get.

When my patients have a bad day or week, I share a favorite quote from Mary Pickford: "Failure lies not in falling down but in *staying* down." Think about that, and consider repeating it to yourself when you feel you have "fallen down" in your weight-loss program, either by overindulging or not exercising (or both).

Anxious about Anxiety?

Anxiety is one of the most common types of psychological symptoms. Feeling worry, fear, and anxiousness is a normal part of human life, but when those feelings interfere with everyday life, it can be a sign of an anxiety disorder. Although some studies have found a link between anxiety and excess weight, others have not. And if there is a connection, we don't really know whether being overweight would cause anxiety, or if anxious people overeat in order to feel better. In my experience, I find that many of my patients suffering from anxiety overeat as a result, and they generally crave dense carbs and high-sugar, high-fat foods.

There are several kinds of anxiety disorders, including generalized anxiety disorder (GAD), obsessive-compulsive disorder (OCD), panic disorder, post-traumatic stress disorder (PTSD), and social anxiety disorder.

Clinical Pearl: *Loosen Up*

I often see all-or-nothing thinking when someone is trying to lose weight for a special event like a wedding or reunion. I remember one patient with disordered eating who wanted to lose 30 pounds in three months for her sister's wedding. She was very strict with herself and followed her diet exactly for the entire three months without allowing herself any flexibility. I tried very hard to get her to relax on occasion and to have a more long-term approach to healthy eating, but she refused because she was fixated on the number on the scale. She did manage to lose 30 pounds in three months and felt great at her sister's wedding, but faced with all those tempting foods, she binged her way through the weekend and found it very hard to get back on track when she returned. She came to see me to lose the 10 pounds that she had regained and 10 more that she still wanted to lose, but I refused to see her until she sought professional help for her disordered eating. ◇

Some of the symptoms of anxiety include frequently feeling anxious, worried, annoyed, irritable, or nervous; having trouble relaxing; feeling restless; and feeling that something terrible might happen.

If anxiety is getting in the way of your day-to-day routine—or if you think it is interfering with your ability to live a healthy lifestyle—talk with your doctor or schedule a consultation with a Doctor on Demand psychologist. Like other psychological disorders, anxiety can be successfully treated with medication and/or therapy.

 SOAP Notes

Stressed Woman Makes Second Attempt at Weight Loss

Kathy is a petite woman in her 30s with metabolic syndrome (high blood sugar, high cholesterol, waist greater than 35 inches, family history of diabetes) who came to see me 10 years ago and lost 32 pounds in just over six months. After six months, her weight loss plateaued and she slowly began to regain weight and stopped coming in to see me. She began seeing me again a few years later after having regained nearly all of her lost weight, but was committed to taking off her excess weight for good. Here is a note from one of her visits the second time around.

Subjective:

Patient is under a lot of stress, not sleeping well, and skipping meals several times per week. Not keeping track of her food consistently. Exercising three times a week (despite my recommendation of five days per week) because she says she hates going to the gym. Reports pants feeling roomier even though scale not moving as quickly as she would like.

Objective:

Weight down 4.6 pounds in past month. Food journal shows frequent meal skipping, especially lunch, and increased intake of dry carbs, including crackers and pita chips in the afternoon and evening.

Assessment and Plan:

1. Inadequate exercise: Aim for goal of exercising five times per week for optimal weight loss. Patient had expressed interest in starting to play tennis again, so I encouraged her to schedule a regular weekly game or two to boost exercise without having to go to the gym any more than necessary. Also encouraged increase in lifestyle exercise such as walking to work and to lunch several times per week. Explained that exercise is important not just for weight loss, but as an excellent way to reduce feelings of stress.

2. Meal skipping: Patient reports no time for lunch on many days, so I encouraged her to stock the fridge at work with precut vegetables, hummus, Greek yogurt, high-fiber/low-sugar fruits (apples, berries), and lean sliced turkey for quick and easy no-prep lunches. I also suggested she bring dinner leftovers to eat for lunch the next day.

3. Excess snacking on dry carbs: I explained that these types of carbs really don't give you a lot of bang for your buck, as they usually do not satisfy hunger effectively (in suggested portions) and are more calorie-dense than other, more-satiating snacks so should be limited as much as possible. Suggested adding a dense carb to dinner (such as quinoa, beans, or barley) to see if that would help with sleep; also started her on a B complex vitamin supplement to help her body combat stress, which can lead to carb cravings. Recommended an occasional glass of wine, which

patient had avoided for months, because it may help her feel less stressed and may make her plan more livable.

Result:

Kathy has lost 44 pounds and has kept it off for several years.

—*Melina B. Jampolis, MD*

Healthy Ways to Relax

If you're struggling with stress—and believe me, as the busy working mother of two little ones, I know what that feels like—think about what changes you can make to reduce stress. Studies show that feeling stressed can contribute to weight gain and interfere with weight loss, so it's smart to make stress reduction part of your healthy-weight plan. Here are a few tips to help you relax.

- **Look at your life.** Before you can reduce stress, you have to understand what's causing it. Take some time to analyze your life and look at what causes tension and anxiety in you. Common stressors include work, family, finances, relationships, world events, health, and busy schedules. If you're the journaling type, start a stress journal.

- **Brainstorm strategies.** Once you identify the sources of your stress, think about strategies that you might be able to use to overcome them. If you're having problems at work, consider setting up a meeting with your boss or a supportive coworker to have a positive discussion about your top-of-mind concerns. If you're having money troubles, consider seeking out a financial advisor, an online money-management program, or even a budget-savvy friend to help you put together a plan to cut spending and pay off debt. If a relationship is causing stress, have a heart-to-heart with the other person, or consider meeting with a counselor or trusted friend who can help smooth things out. If your jam-packed schedule is the problem, try to accept that for a while, you'll have to say no to nonessential activities and set boundaries with friends, family, or colleagues who are asking for more than you can give.

- **Lean on friends.** Spending time with members of your social support network can be a great stress reducer. Friends, supportive family members, neighbors, church or community groups, and online social networks are a great way to connect with others who may be experiencing similar challenges. I find that especially helpful when I get stressed by the trials of being a working mother. It really helps to read or connect with others going through the same situations.

- **Take care of your body.** Exercise, sleep, and eating a healthy diet strengthen your ability to handle stress, so make them a priority.

- **Limit comfort foods.** Turning to sugary, fatty, salty comfort foods may seem like a good idea when you're feeling really stressed, but ultimately they'll just make you feel worse because of the guilt and the subsequent crash in blood sugar that you'll experience after you eat them. Reach for healthier versions of your favorite comfort foods, or keep portions very small. After you successfully push aside a tempting food, focus on how good it feels to triumph over temptation, and how empty you would have felt if you'd given in.

- **Learn relaxation techniques.** Breathing exercises, meditation, prayer, yoga, tai chi, and guided visualization are just a few of the stress-reduction techniques that can really work well. If you don't have time to take a class or join a group that teaches relaxation techniques, consider the many apps, audio recordings, downloads, books, websites, and videos that are now available.

- **Dabble in your passions.** If saying "om" doesn't fit your personality, try to make time for relaxing hobbies or pursuing new interests. Anything that gets your mind off your worries, from drawing to woodworking.

- **Volunteer.** Sometimes, helping others is the best way to help ourselves. Collecting cans for a food drive, walking dogs at your local animal shelter, helping a newcomer learn English, or even making a cash donation to a worthy cause can elicit good feelings that help take the spotlight off our own problems.

- **Sip some tea.** Just taking five minutes out of your day to sit and enjoy a cup of tea can help. Tea contains a chemical called theanine that helps promote relaxation.

Coming Up Next

Changing your behavior is a great way to position yourself for weight-loss success. But your environment is a factor, too. Your family, friends, and coworkers play a dramatic part in how you eat, exercise, and think about weight loss. So does the arrangement of your kitchen and even the size of your plates! By understanding all this, you can maximize your social and physical environment for optimal success. In the next chapter, I'll show you how making some simple changes can boost your chances of meeting your goals, and I'll share some amazing ways to create a physical and social environment that will support you on your weight-loss journey.

CHAPTER 8

—⁂—

Create an Environment That Supports Success

The world around us influences what we eat, how much we eat, whether we exercise, and many of the other choices we make throughout the day that affect weight loss. This influence can be negative or positive—for example, when you go out to dinner your sister may fuss at you because you don't want to split an order of nachos (negative), or she may encourage you to order the garden salad, with a reminder to get the dressing on the side (positive). I'm lucky when it comes to sisters, as mine is a personal trainer who always inspires me to work out even more than usual when I'm with her.

You can maximize your chances of meeting your weight-loss goals by becoming aware of the many environmental influences that shape your reality and by working to shift negatives to positives. You can also make some simple changes in your environment that will help support, rather than sabotage, your good intentions.

Subverting Social Sabotage

We love our friends and family, and assume they want the best for us. But sometimes—especially when it comes to weight loss—our social network actually interferes with our goals, making it harder, rather than easier, to eat right and exercise. You can make sure this doesn't happen by being aware of the potential saboteurs in your life and planning around them.

Family: Beyond the genetic component of obesity, family plays an important social role in your eating. If you have children or a spouse with a sweet

167

tooth who is naturally thin, you are probably constantly confronted with challenging foods in the house. If this is so, consider designating a cabinet or drawer in the fridge or pantry just for them that is off limits for you.

Do your best to get the family on board for healthier meals and ask for their help or support in limiting temptation by having fewer less-healthful options around and going out to restaurants with healthier choices.

You can also have the family help you get more active by suggesting fun ways for the whole family to get moving throughout the week.

Friends: Research shows that friends—especially same-sex friends—have the greatest potential to negatively influence your weight. For this reason, it is especially important to consider their influence on your weight-loss goals.

Being with friends who are overeating or making poor choices makes it more acceptable to do so yourself, and friends who are not watching their weight may encourage you to indulge, urging you to "just relax and have fun" rather than respecting your goals.

You have a few choices when it comes to dealing with these diet saboteur friends: you can avoid them until you feel more in control of your eating, you can have a heart-to-heart with them and ask for their support, or you can suggest non-eating social outings such as going for a walk or to the movies or a museum.

Coworkers: The workplace can be an eating minefield, beginning with breakfast meetings consisting of coffee and donuts to business lunches and break rooms stocked with snack food. Most of us don't have the type of relationship with colleagues that would allow us to feel comfortable discussing weight-loss goals, so the best strategy is to proactively manage your office eating environment. Here are some tips:

- Request healthful food choices (if available) for breakfast meetings, or bring your own meal (fruit, yogurt, or a protein bar are all excellent portable choices).
- For business lunches, volunteer to choose the restaurant and pick one with healthy options. If someone else chooses, look up the menu online beforehand and plan your meal so you won't be tempted just to order what others get.
- If the break room is too tempting, avoid it, especially at high-risk times of day like midafternoon.

~ Stock your desk with snack options for the week, including fruit, single-size servings of nuts, and low-sugar energy bars.

Research on Demand: Is Weight Gain Contagious?

You can't "catch" obesity from others. But a 32-year-long study of over 12,000 people published in the *New England Journal of Medicine* in 2007 found that the spouses, family members, and friends of obese people have a higher likelihood of becoming obese. In fact, having an obese friend or family member appeared to increase an individual's chance of becoming obese by 57 percent. Researchers say that regular contact with obese people changes our ideas about what kind of body type is acceptable.

The bottom line: Don't abandon your overweight friends. Instead, see if you can get them to join you in your quest to lose weight, or at least ask for their support instead of sabotage. When you're with slim friends, pay attention to the choices they make. You may learn some great strategies from them.

The Power of Plates

Mindless eating is eating without paying attention, and it often involves eating more food than we really need or foods we aren't really hungry for. We all eat mindlessly sometimes, but there's hope: becoming more aware of our mindless eating habits helps us change them.

Much of what we know about mindless eating comes from Brian Wansink, PhD. He is the director of the Cornell Food and Brand Lab (www.foodpsychology.cornell.edu) and an expert on eating behavior, nutrition science, and food psychology. He's also the author of two excellent books on the topic, *Mindless Eating: Why We Eat More Than We Think* and *Slim by Design: Mindless Eating Solutions for Everyday Life.*

According to Wansink, mindlessness is a big factor in overeating. "Most of us don't overeat because we're hungry. We overeat because of family and friends, packages and plates, names and numbers, labels and lights, colors and candles, shapes and smells, distractions and distances, cupboards and containers," Wansink says. "Our studies show that the average person makes around 250 decisions about food every day—breakfast or no breakfast? Pop-Tart or bagel? Part of it or all of it? Kitchen or car? Yet out of these 200+ food decisions, most we cannot really explain."

What's more, the tools we use to eat—plates, bowels, and flatware—can also contribute to overeating and mindless eating. Making mindful choices about the eating tools you use can have a pretty dramatic effect on your food intake.

If you would like to learn more about mindless eating, I recommend that you read Wansink's books or check out his website, www.slimbydesign .org. I'll also share some of his tips, which my patients have found extremely helpful. The following suggestions are used with his permission:

- **Replace your 12-inch plate with a 10-inch plate.** Research shows that we tend to over-serve onto larger plates—using the plate size as a guide, we guesstimate portions that are bigger than they should be. And since people tend to consume an average of 92 percent of what they have been served, larger plates lead automatically to larger food intake. A two-inch decrease in plate diameter size—from 12 inches to 10 inches—would result in 22 percent fewer calories being served, but it is not a drastic enough difference for our stomachs to notice.

- **Use smaller bowls.** I also recommend shrinking your bowls. My husband and I started using our toddler's bowls instead of our full-sized bowls for everything from yogurt to chili to cereal, and he lost five pounds without really making any other changes and I effortlessly lost a couple of pounds, too.

- **Slim down your glasses.** With glasses, think thin if you want to be thin. We tend to pour 30 percent more into a wide glass than into a slender one. And don't forget to downsize your wine glass, too. Five ounces of wine in a traditional red wine glass barely fills the bottom, leading many people to pour themselves far more than a single serving. (Save larger glasses for drinking water, which helps to fill you up.)

- **Mini-size your boxes.** The larger the package you pour from, the more you will eat: as much as 20 to 30 percent more for most foods, studies show. To keep serving sizes more reasonable, repackage your jumbo box into smaller resealable bags or washable containers.

- **See it before you eat it.** Put everything you want to eat on a plate or in a bowl before you begin eating meals, desserts, or snacks. Also, instead of eating directly out of a package, bag, or box, put your snack in a separate dish and leave the original container in the kitchen. Taking these steps, you'll likely eat less food.

- **Choose a smaller spoon or eat with chopsticks.** In studies, bigger spoons led to bigger servings. Even nutrition experts served themselves up to 31 percent more food when given a larger serving spoon compared to a smaller spoon. I actually found a set of small silver spoons at a garage sale a few years ago and I love using them for desserts, as it really slows me down and makes my dessert last longer.

- **Keep serving dishes off the table.** Having a full dish of food available makes it more likely we'll take more; keeping serving dishes off the table gives us a chance to ask ourselves if we're really hungry before we take more food. The exception to this rule is salad and vegetables: having them on the table can encourage you and your family to eat more of them.

Research on Demand: Smaller Packages, Less Eating

I am a huge fan of 100-calorie packaging (especially nuts). In my experience, when people have a 100-calorie package of food, they're much less likely to overeat than if they're trying to guess calories while they're eating. A 2011 study by Brian Wansink and his colleagues published in the journal *Obesity* bears this out. They gathered two groups of volunteers and gave them crackers to snack on while watching TV. All of the volunteers received 400 calories worth of crackers, but the packaging differed: one group was given four 100-calorie packs, and the other group received one 400-calorie pack. It turned out that on average, study participants who were given four 100-calorie packs ate 25.2 percent (75 calories) less than those who ate from the bigger package. The results were even more dramatic among overweight people: their cracker intake decreased by 54.1 percent when eating from 100-calorie packs.

The bottom line: Choose 100-calorie packaging for nuts, cheese, crackers, and any other foods you're tempted to overeat. If you prefer to avoid the extra packaging or premium prices on these prepackaged foods, portion them out from a larger container using small bags or reusable containers. By reading labels and using measuring spoons or a small scale, you can determine how much food makes up a 100-calorie serving.

Mindful by Design

Unless you live alone, it's probably impossible to get rid of every tempting or unhealthy food in your house, so a little creative kitchen arranging can go a long way toward weight-loss success. You've probably heard the expression "out of sight, out of mind." This definitely applies to food. *Where* you put groceries in your kitchen can actually have a significant impact on what you eat. I always suggest that patients place healthier food at eye level or in visible locations in the pantry, refrigerator, and freezer, and keep more tempting, less healthy foods out of sight. For example:

- Keep the frozen broccoli and chicken breasts at eye level in your freezer and the ice cream sandwiches on the lowest shelf or, even better, in a freezer drawer.
- Store soups and whole grains at eye level in the pantry and crackers and cookies on higher shelves (and limit the variety of less healthful foods to make it even easier for you to control calories effortlessly).
- Place fruit in a bowl on the counter rather than in a drawer in the refrigerator.
- If you must have a cookie jar for your kids, get an opaque container so you don't have to stare down the chocolate chip cookies every time you go in the kitchen.

One of my patients reorganized her kitchen and found that she actually completely forgot about tempting treats when they were out of sight and was surprised to find an untouched box of her favorite salty snacks months later when she was cleaning out her cabinets. Another patient has her husband hide her chocolate-covered almonds and dole them out to her one at a time when she needs a little treat.

Mindless eating can lead you to eat hundreds of extra calories every day. By making changes in your environment—some as simple as using a smaller plate or placing a fruit bowl on your counter—you can take away some of the mindless eating triggers that have interfered with weight-loss success.

Research on Demand: Be Mindful of Calories

Although I don't focus on calorie counting in the Doctor on Demand Diet, I do suggest that you pay attention to calorie listings on food labels, menus, and signs, because they can encourage mindfulness and can help you to be aware of what you're eating. This strategy is reinforced by a study published in 2014 in the journal *Obesity*. In the study, researchers measured the impact of menus in a college cafeteria that listed the calorie contents of food. They found that when calorie counts were listed, students did not gain weight during the school year, but when calorie counts were not listed, students gained an average of nearly eight pounds.

The bottom line: Don't get obsessed with calories, but definitely be mindful and pay attention to calorie counts on packages, signs, and menus. Doing so may help you eat less and lose more.

Coming Up Next

It's one thing to be able to follow your diet and exercise plans when you're at home. But it's quite another to be able to stick to them when you're out in the world—in restaurants, at work, at parties, or while traveling. Sure, it's a challenge, but you can do it! All it takes is some awareness of what to expect and some smart planning so that you're ready to handle just about any situation that comes along. In the next chapter, you'll learn everything you need to know to make smart food and fitness choices when you're away from home.

CHAPTER 9

—◊◊◊—

Eating in the Real World

For most of my patients, sticking with their healthy eating plan is relatively easy when they're at home. Sure, they have temptations, but in general, once they figure out what to eat and how big their portions should be, they can do a good job staying on track when they're preparing their own food in their own homes.

All that can change when they leave their kitchens behind and go out into the world—to work, restaurants, and other people's homes, as well as while traveling. More challenges and less control is an equation that makes smart eating much more difficult. When you're out in the world, not only must you deal with temptations at work—I'm talking about you, pastry tray at the weekly budget meeting—but you must also navigate your way through restaurant menus, buffet tables, salad bars, and grab-and-go food displays whenever you're out on the town. Even stores that sell clothing, electronics, and hardware often have candy and soda for sale near the cash registers.

This is an issue that has to be addressed, because most of us spend large chunks of time away from our homes at mealtimes. On average, adults in America eat five of their 21 weekly meals in restaurants; almost half of our weekly food budgets are spent on restaurant meals. Add in all the times we eat in other people's homes, at our workplaces, or on the road, and you end up with a huge challenge.

Weekends and holiday celebrations can also make it harder to stay on track. People who do perfectly well following their diets Monday through Friday often struggle with it on Saturdays and Sundays. And we all know how tough it can be to avoid tempting foods at holiday parties, family gatherings, and even summer barbecues.

Fortunately, you can meet all of the challenges that the real world throws in your path. There are many ways to eat smart when you're away from home and on weekends and holidays. By planning ahead and learning some simple real-world eating strategies, you can exercise more control over your away-from-home eating experiences.

In this chapter, I'll share some of my favorite, most successful strategies. I'll also give you some specific recommendations for foods you can order in various kinds of restaurants. By following them, you'll boost your chances of eating right and meeting your weight-loss goals.

A Menu of Choices:
Strategies for Eating in Restaurants

For most of us, eating in restaurants is just part of life—we simply don't live in a way that allows us to eat made-at-home meals every day. Eating out also has an important social and, for some people, business function. While it is easier to lose weight by not eating out, this is simply not realistic for the majority of people (including myself).

Restaurants, food manufacturers, and even convenience stores are responding to consumers' desire to have healthy, lower-calorie, lower-fat, higher-fiber choices on menus and shelves. The trick is to know how to order a meal that fits your needs. Here are some strategies that have worked for my patients (and me).

Do your homework. Many of my patients like to look up restaurant menus online ahead of time to figure out the best options and plan their day accordingly. You can also look up the nutrition stats at fast-food and fast-casual restaurants to figure out what works best with your eating plan.

Bypass bread. Ask the waiter not to bring it or to take it away. If your dining partners want bread, keep the basket on their side of the table.

Choose lean protein. Grilled chicken or fish are good options. For sides, request two orders of veggies without sauce or butter (or get the sauce on the side so you can apply just a teaspoon or two). In a steakhouse, select leaner cuts, like filet mignon, instead of fattier cuts such as prime rib or porterhouse.

Control your portion size. Split meals, or plan (and follow through) to take half home for lunch the next day.

Read the fine print. Opt for dishes with names that include words like *steamed, broiled, roasted, grilled,* and *poached* instead of *fried, crispy, breaded,* and *sautéed.* But remember that even simply cooked foods can be drizzled with fat; tell your waiter you want your protein "naked." Order salad dressing and all sauces on the side.

Go beyond entrées. Consider ordering an appetizer or an appetizer and a salad as your entrée, especially if you are having a cocktail or plan on sharing a little dessert. Often, salads can be ordered with a piece of fish or chicken on top.

Choose dense carbs wisely. If you have a little bread, don't eat the rice or potato too! If you decide to have a side of pasta, skip the bread.

When in doubt, ask. If you can't figure out what a particular dish is made of, ask your waiter. If he or she doesn't know, skip it. It's better to play it safe and not risk sabotaging your diet. It's also important to ask about sides—I can't tell you how many times my husband has ordered something that he did not realize came with fries. He doesn't intend to eat them, but once they are sitting in front of him, they can be very hard to resist.

Don't drink your calories. Skip the lemonade, sweet tea, juice, and soda, and limit alcohol. You are already probably having more calories by eating out, so don't make things worse with less-filling liquid calories.

Be rational about dessert. If you budgeted dessert into your day, and the selections really look good, just eat a few bites, or split dessert with a friend. Don't waste calories on the vanilla ice cream you could have anytime or a mediocre apple tart.

Do your best. Try to make the smartest choices possible, and plan to make up for any indulgences the next day with a little more exercise or a little less fat or dry carbs.

Plan post-meal exercise. Go for a walk in the neighborhood or dancing at a club after your meal.

Clinical Pearl: *Best Morning Meals*

When eating out for breakfast or brunch, eggs are a good choice, because they're high in protein and omelets can be ordered with vegetables. Save calories by skipping the cheese, choosing ham or turkey bacon rather than regular bacon or sausage, and asking that your eggs be prepared with minimal or no added fat. (Have you ever watched how much oil they use to make omelets at an omelet bar? It's often several tablespoons, so it's important to ask for oil spray or minimal oil if possible.) Request fresh fruit as a side (or whole-grain toast if available), and stay away from biscuits, scones, muffins, and coffee cake, which are typically incredibly high in fat and calories. ◇

Best Choices at Ethnic Restaurants

When you move beyond classic American bistro food, it can be tricky to figure out what to order. Here's a guide for some popular ethnic fare.

Mexican

- Use moderation when eating guacamole. Choose salsa instead. Even though guacamole is a fantastic source of healthy fats, the calories can add up fast. Save guacamole and avocadoes for times when you are eating a lighter-in-calorie meal or snack.

- Avoid refried beans, as they are cooked in lard, added fats, and salt. Choose fresh black beans as an alternative.

- If you like soup, choose a cup of black bean soup or tortilla soup with little or no cheese.

- Instead of quesadillas, order chicken or shrimp fajitas or soft tacos with whole-wheat or corn tortillas. Skip the cheese, and have a little guacamole and lots of salsa.

- If you order a taco salad, pass up the fried shell in which the salad is served. Ask the kitchen to leave off the cheese and serve the dressing on the side. If there are any additions such as sour cream, avocado, and refried beans, opt out or ask for them on the side. Make sure to exercise portion control. Select grilled meats (beef, chicken, pork, or fish) instead of carnitas (fried pork) or chorizo (sausage), which are less healthful options.

- Order enchiladas with green or red sauce, not cream sauce. And stick with chicken instead of cheese or beef.

- Stay away from the chip basket. You probably can't eat "just a few."

- Skip the margarita. Most have well over 300 calories of sugar and alcohol. If you must have a cocktail, have a beer or ask for a "skinny margarita," which consists of tequila with lime juice only and club soda.

Italian

- Try not to get pasta as an entrée. Have it on the side or as a "primi" plate, as they do in Italy. If you have bread, skip the pasta, and vice versa.

- Start with a bowl of minestrone soup, a green salad, or a tomato/mozzarella appetizer.

- Avoid breaded dishes like parmigiana; opt for marsala or marinara instead.

- Skip the fatty sauces, like Alfredo, carbonara, or cream, which can add hundreds of calories. Watch the pesto, too—even though it is healthier, it is not calorie-free.

- Ask for a side of veggies instead of pasta, if possible.

- Grilled or broiled chicken and fish are healthy choices. Make sure to avoid buttered sides. Request your vegetable sides freshly steamed, with no added butter or sauces.

Chinese

- Start with wonton, hot and sour, or egg drop soup and avoid other appetizers

- Skip the white or fried rice; ask for brown rice.

- Ask for dry wok, when possible.

- Experiment with Chinese veggies, and opt for chicken, tofu, or seafood, as the red meat can be quite fatty.

- Pick a chicken, shrimp, or vegetable dish rather than a noodle or rice dish, which tend to be pretty skimpy on the vegetables and heavy on the sodium and fat.
- Avoid sweet-and-sour or fried dishes.
- Order an entrée that is stir-fried or steamed.
- Watch the nuts in dishes; they can add up to 1/2 cup or more (350 or more calories).

Thai

- Avoid coconut and peanut sauces (or order on the side). Opt for oyster or black bean sauces instead.
- Order any entrée with veggies, or get a side of veggies.
- Stick with chicken, seafood, or tofu, all lower-fat options.
- Consider chicken/tofu/shrimp satay as an appetizer, or a cucumber salad.
- Drink regular brewed tea or water. Skip the Thai tea; it's pure sugar and cream.
- Try the curry, and limit the MSG. Ask the chef to prepare meals with minimal "low sodium" soy sauce. Curries are a blend of spices, and the sauces they are mixed in can be fatty. Make sure to ask how the curries are prepared and choose the best possible choice of sauce per recommendations. Avoid coconut- or cream-based curries, which are calorie bombshells.

Japanese

- Start with miso soup, plain edamame (soy beans), or salad with a teaspoon or two of non-cream-based dressing.
- Skip tempura (and any rolls with tempura).
- Ask for "light rice" for rolls, which can reduce dense carbs. Select brown rice if available.
- Sushi: four pieces of sushi = approximately 1/2 cup rice (one dense carb), so limit to eight pieces, *maximum.*
- Watch higher-fat ingredients in rolls, such as cream cheese, avocado, and mayo in spicy tuna or crab; they add hundreds of calories.
- Sashimi is a great choice.

French

- ❧ Simple is better—if it sounds complicated, it is probably not good for your diet.

- ❧ Skip the sauces and preparation methods that are super high in fat, such as crème, au gratin, au beurre (which means butter), hollandaise, and more.

- ❧ Limit the amount of cheese or avoid all together.

- ❧ Dips and cream-based soups can add many extra calories, so avoid as best as possible.

Indian

- ❧ Tandoori dishes are a good low-fat choice, with lots of spices.

- ❧ Choose multiple vegetable (curry) and lentil dishes.

- ❧ Avoid fried dishes and coconut sauces.

- ❧ If a menu descriptor uses the words "paneer," "ghee," or "malai," then avoid these dishes or have just a taste of someone else's. Paneers are high-fat cheese, ghee is butter, and malai is milk.

- ❧ Limit the nan; once you start eating this delicious Indian bread, it may be hard to stop.

- ❧ Limit or avoid the basmati rice; calories can add up fast, with a single cup containing 200 calories or more.

- ❧ Always ask about the dish if you are unsure. If you don't know what a word means, ask before ordering; this way your waitstaff can help guide you toward healthier options.

Fitting in Fast Food

While many obesity experts blame fast food for the country's rising obesity epidemic, our hectic lifestyles and limited budgets often make fast food unavoidable. While I am in no way advocating fast food, I do realize that many people who are trying to lose weight rely on fast-food and fast-casual restaurants as an eating option.

If you're careful, you can get a decent meal at many fast-food places, provided you educate yourself on the available menu items, choose carefully, and pay attention to portion sizes. If you eat fast food regularly, make sure the rest of your diet includes lots of fresh vegetables, fruits, and whole grains.

Here are some other ways to fit fast food into the Doctor on Demand plan:

- Avoid large, jumbo, or supersize *anything*. Don't be lured in by lower prices: the extra calories, sugar, salt, fat, and associated health risks of these humongous portions are not worth the dollar you save.

- Skip fried or breaded sandwiches. Instead choose broiled or grilled options, such as grilled chicken.

- Hold the cheese, creamy or honey sauces, and mayo, which add hundreds of calories. Stick with mustard, ketchup, hot sauce— even BBQ sauce in small amounts is OK.

- Avoid regular soda and sugary juice drinks, including lemonade and sweet teas.

- Leave off the bun—or just eat half. And stay away from high-fat breads, such as croissants and biscuits, which add a surprising amount of calories and fat.

- Limit fast food if you have high blood pressure, because it is much higher in salt (even salads) than most other types of food.

- When ordering a salad, ask for dressing on the side. Even the low-fat version can add a hundred calories in some cases. To minimize how much dressing you eat, dip your fork in the dressing, and then spear the vegetables. And avoid high-fat or high-calorie toppings, such as bacon, cheese, tortilla chips, croutons, and noodles.

- In a pizza place, stick with mainly veggie toppings (chicken and ham/pineapple are OK, too). Ask for light cheese if possible, or take a bit off, and choose a whole-wheat or thin crust if it's available. Avoid pesto pizza, because it can be very high in fat and calories.

The Best Fast-Food Choices by Restaurant

Burger King

- Hamburger
- Chicken Whopper (*no* mayo)
- BK Veggie Burger (*no* mayo; eat only 1/2 bun)
- BBQ, sweet and sour sauce (all other sauces double the calories or more)
- Side Garden Salad
- Chicken Salad (get dressing on the side; even fat free = 70 calories)

Carl's Jr.

- Charbroiled BBQ Chicken Sandwich
- Charbroiled Chicken Salad-to-Go
- Garden Salad-to-Go: fat-free Italian or dressing on the side
- Hawaiian Grilled Chicken Salad (ask for dressing on the side and lightly drizzle on a teaspoon or two)

Chipotle

- Salads here are a great option (no tortilla); chicken is best, but steak is pretty good, too; get black beans or pinto beans, no rice, salsa (as dressing), fajita vegetables; 1/2 serving of guacamole is optional; skip the cheese

Denny's

- Grilled Chicken Dinner
- Vegetable Beef or Chicken Noodle Soup
- Garden Deluxe Salad with chicken breast, turkey, or ham
- Side Garden Salad
- Eggs and English muffin or toast (dry—you can always add a little butter or jam)
- Healthier sides = carrots in honey glaze, green beans with bacon, sliced tomato, cottage cheese, applesauce

Domino's Pizza

- Cheese, grilled chicken, or vegetable toppings are best
- Always start with large salad with dressing on the side
- Ask for light cheese, and stick with thin crust

Jack in the Box

- Chicken Fajita Pita (hold cheese)
- Breakfast Jack
- Chicken Sandwich (no cheese; no mayo)
- Asian Chicken Salad; skip the crispy wontons
- Chicken Caesar Salad (low-fat balsamic dressing OK)
- Side Salad
- Low-fat Herb Mayo

KFC

- Caesar Salad, no dressing, no croutons
- Honey BBQ Sandwich, side of green beans
- Tender Roast Sandwich (get hot sauce instead of regular sauce)
- Corn on the cob (small)

McDonald's

- Hamburger
- English Muffin and 2 Scrambled Eggs (with coffee or water, not juice)
- Egg McMuffin (hold the cheese)
- Fruit 'n Yogurt Parfait
- Chicken McGrill; no mayo (ask for BBQ or hot mustard sauce packet instead)
- Premium Grilled Chicken Caesar with reduced-fat dressing
- Vanilla Reduced-Fat Ice Cream Cone (my favorite occasional treat)
- Grilled Chicken Bacon Ranch (Drizzle lightly with Newman's Own Low-Fat Balsamic Vinaigrette)

- Premium Southwest Salad with Grilled Chicken (avoid the cheese and tortilla strips; drizzle lightly with lime or light balsamic dressing)
- Side Salad

Panda Express
(If you have high blood pressure, limit Chinese fast food, as most choices are loaded with sodium.)

- Black Pepper Chicken
- Chicken with Mushrooms
- Chicken with String Beans
- Beef with Broccoli or String Beans
- Mixed Vegetables
- Hot and Sour Soup
- Low-sodium soy sauce (limit, as meals already cooked in this), hot mustard sauce, or hot sauce

Panera Bread

- Lower-carb breads (Italian, Pumpkin) better option, or whole-grain baguette or loaf
- Good choice of low-fat soups, including Chicken Noodle, Vegetarian Black Bean, Moroccan Lentil, Garden Vegetable
- Asian Sesame Chicken Salad, Grilled Chicken Caesar (ask for the cheese on the side), Fandango Salad (fat-free poppy seed or fat-free raspberry dressing, reduced-sugar Asian Sesame Vinaigrette); request dressings on the side and drizzle lightly for optimal portion control
- Fresh Fruit Cup

Subway

- Choose any 6-inch sandwich with 6 grams of fat (Chicken, Roast Beef, Turkey, Veggie Delite) on a whole-wheat low-carb wrap instead of bread; skip the oil, mayo, and cheese, or get one of the new lower fat mini subs with a side salad
- Grilled Chicken and Baby Spinach Salad with no croutons or cheese

- Subway Club Salad
- Veggie Delite Salad
- Kraft Fat-Free Italian Dressing or any other on the side
- Soups (1 cup): Minestrone, Roasted Chicken Noodle (high salt)
- Breakfast Sandwich on Deli Round (topless, no cheese)

Taco Bell

- Order items "Fresco" = salsa in place of cheese and sauce
- Fiesta or Express Taco Salad without shell or Red Strips
- Fresco Chicken Taco (soft or crunchy*)
- Fresco Grilled Steak Taco (soft or crunchy*)

   * The crunchy taco has less salt if you are watching salt intake.

Wendy's

- Ultimate Chicken Grill Sandwich (high salt, eat 1/2 bun)
- Jr. Burger (eat 1/2 bun)
- Small chili without cheese (adds 70 calories)
- Grilled chicken with honey mustard dressing (reduced fat) or no dressing
- Spring Mix Salad (pecans OK, but count as fat)
- Asian Chicken half salad (skip crispy noodles; almonds OK, but count as fat)
- Side Salad or Caesar Side Salad with no croutons; drizzle lightly with the lemon garlic Caesar dressing
- Apple Pecan Chicken, half size

Research on Demand: A Good Reason to Eat at Home

On days when adults eat at restaurants (either fast-food or full-service), they consume about 200 more calories than they do on days they eat at home, according to a 2014 study published in *Public Health Nutrition*. The study also found that eating at restaurants led to increases in the intake of sugar, sodium, and saturated fat. Other studies have found that the more often people eat in restaurants, the more likely they are to gain weight over time; healthy-weight people who eat in restaurants more frequently have a higher chance of becoming overweight or obese than those who eat in restaurants less often.

The bottom line: Try not to eat in restaurants too frequently; when you do, eat mindfully, choosing foods that fit into your plan. Even though this study found that people eat 200 extra calories in restaurants, my experience is that the increased intake is, for many of my patients, much higher.

TGIF: *Making a Game Plan for Weekends*

When I worked in San Francisco, my office was located less than an hour from wine country. Many of my patients worked in high-stress jobs during the week and loved to relax on weekends in Napa Valley or Sonoma. This relaxation usually involved amazing wine and great food, both of which could wreak havoc on their diets. While I would never discourage patients from enjoying themselves in one of the most beautiful areas in the country, I spent a lot of time helping them figure out ways to minimize the damage that indulgent weekend eating and drinking could do to their diets. But our work paid off: even in wine country, it's possible to make choices that can enhance weekend fun without destroying the progress made during the week.

I know that weekends can be challenging when you are trying to lose or maintain weight. I hear this story on a regular basis: "I've worked hard all week, exercised regularly, planned my meals and snacks, finished that big project at work, drove the kids to and from all of their activities, and now I feel I *deserve* to loosen up a little over the weekend. How much harm can I really do in two and a half days?"

A *lot*. An extra 250 calories per day (the equivalent of one glass of wine and a small cookie) on Friday, Saturday, and Sunday can add up to a 13-pound weight gain per year, or prevent a 13-pound weight loss, if consumed on a regular basis.

What does this mean to you? While there is room for occasional indulgences, helping to prevent feelings of deprivation and cravings, the key is *keeping* them occasional—and moderate. Don't "let go" entirely on weekends. If you do, you will constantly be taking two steps forward and one—or two—steps back. This can slow your progress considerably and be very discouraging over the long term.

So, what can you do to prevent your weekends from sabotaging all your Monday through Friday progress? Here's my advice:

Relax by moving. We all like to chill out on the weekends, but that doesn't mean putting your feet up for two days. Exercise is one of the most relaxing activities you can engage in. I'm always astonished when my patients tell me they didn't exercise at all over the weekend because they "just wanted to relax." Weekends are the best time to exercise, because you probably have more time over the weekend than during the week. Motivate yourself to do more activity, not less, over the weekend. Wear a step counter and see how many steps you can accumulate on weekend days. Challenge yourself to increase your total by a few hundred steps each weekend.

Involve your family. Take your family on a long hike or bike ride, or take up a new sport as a family. I remember going to tennis camp as a kid and having a blast, and afterward we all had a fun activity to do together. Instead of thinking of exercise as a chore to be completed over the weekend, make it fun! You can also replace your Saturday night family movie with a crazy '80s dance party (leg warmers and neon optional). Or fire up the Wii fitness device and challenge the neighbors to an interfamily fitness contest. During warmer months, set up an obstacle course in your backyard or at a local park.

Aim to maintain. Many of my patients find it easier to approach weekends with the goal of maintaining their weight rather than being strict in their effort to lose weight. Though consistency is key, finding the balance between consistency and livability is essential. If you enjoy having dessert or an extra glass of wine on weekends, or perhaps a less restrictive brunch, go ahead. Just make sure that you don't go completely overboard and have six cocktails, a large slice of cheesecake, and French toast loaded with syrup the next day. I don't recommend taking a "day off" or even an entire meal "off" as some diets recommend, but a planned indulgence will not interfere significantly with your weight loss in the short or long term and may even help you mentally stay on track.

Think before you drink. Research suggests that weekend calories often come from alcohol, so it makes sense to limit alcohol if you are trying to lose weight. This is smart not just because alcohol contains calories, but because it may stimulate appetite in some people and can reduce your willpower. Healthy choices seem a lot less appealing after a couple glasses of wine.

Make Mine a Vodka Soda Tall

When you opt to have an alcoholic beverage, a "vodka soda tall" is a good choice—in fact, it's my preferred drink. I recommend it because you can make it big enough to last a long time.

A typical glass of wine is five ounces (120 calories), although restaurants often pour more, and at home, because of the size of most wine glasses, a glass of wine can weigh in at eight or more ounces. (Try pouring five ounces of water into one of your wine glasses, then pour it into a measuring cup and see how close you got to five ounces.)

When you order a vodka soda tall, you get a tall glass with a serving of vodka and lots of calorie-free seltzer. Flavored vodka is fine if there's no added sugar, or you can squeeze in fresh lime. For about the same number of calories (and alcohol content) as a little glass of wine, you get a big drink that you can sip on for at least a few rounds. If you're not a fan of vodka, here are a few more higher-volume, lower-calorie options:

- Rum and diet cola
- White wine spritzer (add equal parts wine and club soda to double your portion of wine without doubling calories)
- Vodka soda with a splash of cranberry, 7-Up, or tonic water and a twist of lime (this adds a little more flavor without adding too many more calories)
- Skinny margarita (many restaurants now offer these lower-calorie options made with tequila, club soda, and fresh lime juice—you can add in a packet of no-calorie sweetener if you like)
- Gin and diet tonic (you probably can't find diet tonic water at most bars, but you can easily make this at home)
- Scotch and soda, tall

Some of my patients prefer to eliminate alcohol entirely while they are trying to lose weight, even on Phase 3 of the plan. Others cut back, or just choose to drink when they feel it would be most enjoyable. Choose whatever strategy works best for you. If you do imbibe, consider reducing your intake of dense carbs or fat to make up for it.

Clinical Pearl: *Veggie Dip Tip*

For many of my patients, a veggie platter is their go-to party food and potluck donation. Start with lots of raw carrots, peppers, radishes, celery, broccoli, cherry tomatoes, and other veggies. As for dip, guacamole is a delicious source of healthy fat, but it's also high in calories. You can make a lighter version by mixing equal parts salsa or pico de gallo with premade guacamole or mashed avocado—this cuts calories almost in half by adding lower-calorie vegetables to the mix. You can also slash calories by making dips with low-fat or nonfat sour cream or substituting low-fat Greek yogurt. You'll never notice the difference flavor wise, I promise. The Greek Yogurt Hummus and the Green Goddess-Style Yogurt Dip in the recipe section are healthful and tasty options. ◇

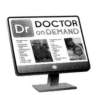 **Research on Demand:**
Weekday Cycling Works

It's normal for people to gain a bit of weight on weekends and then lose it during the week, according to a 2014 study published in the journal *Obesity Facts*. In the study, researchers asked a group of subjects to record their weight every day. Results showed that subjects weighed the most on Sundays and Mondays, but their weight decreased during the week, with Friday being, on average, their lightest day. The study also found that this "rhythmic compensation pattern" was strongest among people who had lost weight or maintained a steady weight during the study and weakest in those who slowly gained weight, suggesting that it is a strategy for successful weight loss and maintenance.

The bottom line: Compensating during the week for weekend splurges can be a helpful way to meet weight-loss goals over time. In the Doctor on Demand Diet, this is built into the plan in Phase 3, which recommends Diet-Cycling one to two days per week (or more if necessary). It doesn't mean you can go crazy on weekends, but it can make space for a glass of wine or few bites of dessert.

Holidays: How to Have a Merry, Gain-Free Season

Holidays are tough for people who are trying to lose weight or maintain weight loss. The end-of-the-year holiday season that starts with Halloween, continues through Thanksgiving, Hanukah, Christmas, and Kwanza, and wraps up with New Year's Eve/Day is a major danger zone studded with candy, cookies, cocktails, and a huge buffet of other temptations.

Studies have shown that while the average American gains only a pound or two between Thanksgiving and New Year's, those with weight problems often gain 5 to 10 pounds. But don't despair. Many of my patients have successfully maintained their weight over the holidays and a rare few have even lost weight.

I don't expect you to follow your eating plan perfectly during the holidays—there's just too much temptation. But you can make better choices and trade-offs that will allow you to celebrate without ruining months of hard work.

I encourage you to focus on maintenance during December since it is such a challenging time of year, with so much temptation and so many time demands. As always, the key to success is planning. Knowing what you're up against and brainstorming a strategy that fits your life will allow you to get through holidays with minimal weight gain. Here are some tips that have worked well with my patients:

Write a "holiday mission statement" for food and exercise. Spend some time analyzing past holiday eating experiences. Ask yourself how much stuffing, pie, cakes, cookies, bread, and chocolate you have eaten during past holidays. How did all that eating make you feel? How do you want to feel this year? Do you really need more of everything? Using visualization, write about how you will feel in January if you step on the scale and the number on it is (a) too high, (b) exactly the same as it was in October, or (c) lower than before the holidays. Use these feelings to help you craft a "holiday mission statement" that sets out exactly how you want to handle holiday food and exercise. Set realistic goals, put them in writing, and check back often. Being mindful is better than just gliding through the holiday season vaguely hoping that things will work out when you get on the scale in January.

Eat before you party. Starving yourself before a holiday event is a recipe for overeating. Instead, take the edge off your hunger with a small (100 to

150 calories) protein-based, high-fiber snack or mini-meal (Greek yogurt with 1/2 cup of fresh berries or high-fiber cereal, one snack-size smoothie, or half a turkey sandwich on whole-grain bread) and drink a large glass of water before heading out the door to help you minimize indulgences and resist temptation more easily. If you plan to drink alcohol, you may want to include a little fat in your snack, such as string cheese or some nuts, because fat will slow down the absorption of alcohol into your bloodstream.

Bring your own food. To make sure there's something healthy for you to eat, bring along an appetizer (for example, a veggie tray with a low-fat dip) or dessert (such as a fresh fruit platter with the Honey Ricotta Crunch recipe featured in this book).

Drink smart. All alcohol is filled with empty calories, but holiday drinks and cocktails can be even worse than the average glass of wine. For example, one cup of the average eggnog, a Christmas favorite, has 300 calories and 22 grams of fat. If you love these once-a-year drinks, go ahead and have a few sips, but try to stick to lower-calorie drinks, such as champagne, white wine spritzers, unsweetened spiced or mint teas, holiday sangria, skinny holiday punch (make it with reduced-calorie juices or punch mix and dilute calories even more with sparkling water), or sparkling water with a festive fruit garnish.

Schedule exercise first. The holiday season is busy, and even the most devoted gym buff may find it difficult to find time to exercise. That's why I urge you to schedule your workouts weeks in advance, writing them in ink in your datebook (or in bold in your electronic planner) and working in all your holiday commitments—parties, shopping trips, and celebrations—around your exercise schedule. If you wait until you have free time, you'll never exercise, because free time is such a rare commodity during the holidays. If at all possible, look for ways to increase your exercise during the holiday season, because it will help prevent weight gain. Go back to chapter 5 and reread my suggestions for working activity into everyday life, because during the holidays, you need every step you can manage. In addition to your usual workouts, plan fun, active ways to spend time with family and friends. Go for a walk before or after a holiday meal, plan a family hike or snowshoeing party, organize a family

Clinical Pearl: *Be Choosy with Holiday Foods*

As you choose which holiday foods to enjoy and which to pass up, differentiate between truly special holiday foods (your grandmother's once-a-year pumpkin cheesecake or your husband's secret-recipe eggnog) and year-round foods that are simply marketed to take advantage of the holidays (a classic example of this is simply changing the color of candy wrappers). And don't waste calories on the fillers (rolls, chips, cheese, crackers) that are available any time of year.

dance contest after dinner, volunteer to wash dishes or clean the house before or after your family's holiday get-togethers. If after-work holiday parties interfere with exercise, take a walk at lunch or before work. Do anything you can to burn more calories.

Make mindful trade-offs. If you indulge in holiday treats, do so mindfully, and make smart trade-offs. Skip wine at one party, and skip dessert at another. If you have a little bread or pasta, try to limit yourself to only one glass of wine instead of two. Choose just your favorites, and skip the rest.

Use Diet-Cycling to make up for slips. If you've reached the Cycle for Success phase of the Doctor on Demand Diet, use it strategically during the holidays. I always try to sneak in a cycling day or two each week during the holidays on the days that I don't have social plans.

Dress the part. Don't wear loose-fitting "eating clothes" to a party or dinner. This may sound ridiculous, but if your clothes have plenty of room for expansion, you may not realize how stuffed you are getting. Any tactic you can use to get through the holidays without gaining 10 pounds is worth trying, right?

Don't be sidetracked by buffets. Potluck suppers, buffet-style party food, and other serve-yourself arrangements can be a land mine for people trying to lose weight or maintain weight loss. Unfortunately, these all-you-can-eat spreads are a frequent guest at parties and get-togethers throughout

Clinical Pearl: *Weighing In on Holidays*

During the holiday season, get on the scale at least once a week to keep yourself from veering too far off track. Many of my patients avoid the scale completely when they aren't paying attention to their diet and ignore the fact that their favorite pair of pants is getting tighter every day. It's also useful to keep a food journal during the holiday months so you can try to balance out the frequent splurges with lower-calorie meals. ◇

the year. You can survive buffet tables by keeping some of the following strategies in mind:

- **Survey your options.** Before starting to serve yourself, look at all your choices. This allows you to budget your calories more effectively by deciding ahead of time which foods you're going to fill up on (salad, lean protein), which foods you're going to skip, and which foods you're going to splurge a little on. (I always do this year round!)

- **Bring your own dish.** Your hosts will thank you for your generosity, and you'll be making sure there's at least one healthy, low-calorie option on the table.

- **Get away from the table.** After making your choices, move away from the food table for the rest of the night. The farther away you are, the less tempted you will be to go back for more. Believe me, proximity to food matters. Research also shows that facing away from the buffet can help, too.

- **Have a little bit of something special.** Completely depriving yourself may backfire.

What a Trip: Stay on Track While Seeing the World

Vacation and travel are two of the most challenging circumstances for people trying to lose weight or maintain weight loss. The lack of routine and structure can easily derail even the most dedicated nutrition and exercise plan.

For most people, vacations and business travel can easily lead to weight gain, unless perhaps you are trekking in Nepal. Be realistic about weight and travel expectations. Trying to lose weight while on vacation may be too much to expect, but it's realistic to set a goal of having the number on the scale be the same when you arrive home as it was when you departed.

Whether you are traveling for business or pleasure, it is important to plan ahead and try to adopt some of the following strategies.

Skip the starvation scenario. I strongly discourage cutting calories drastically to lose extra weight prior to vacations. This may slow your metabolism and cause quick weight gain when you start eating normally during your trip. It also causes you to begin your trip feeling deprived, and can lead to overeating while you're away.

Move every chance you get. Instead of sitting at the airport, grab your wheeled suitcase and do laps around the terminal. At your destination, walk instead of taking a cab, and fill your itinerary with action-packed activities. Swim, snorkel, go for walks after dinner, bike on country roads, go dancing, or shop. You don't have to frequent the hotel gym in Hawaii or Paris, but make a conscious effort to do more lifestyle-based activities. If you are traveling on business, consider staying at a hotel that has in-room fitness options or a gym. Many hotels now cater to fitness-minded business travelers. Or pack an exercise band and jump rope in your suitcase and do a few exercises and stretches at night.

Plan an active vacation. Activity-based trips can be tremendously enjoyable. Many of my patients have gone on hiking or biking trips to keep up their healthy habits or spent a week at a tennis camp instead of lying on the beach. You feel much better about enjoying a delicious dinner and a glass of wine when you've been hiking all day!

Be prepared. Don't allow yourself to get too hungry—always have healthy snacks such as nuts, protein bars, or fruit in your bag. If your hotel has a refrigerator, stock up at a local market on cottage cheese, string cheese, yogurt, hummus, precut veggies, and fruit for small meals and snacks. Or bring fruit, veggies, or nuts to the pool or sightseeing. One of my patients ships a box of healthy food ahead every time she visits her mother in South America to make sure she always has healthy choices to balance out the heavier food her family often cooks, and Carlos, the busy traveling executive whom I mentioned earlier, takes a mini-blender and protein shake packets on every trip.

Choose your splurges carefully. Just as brightly wrapped candies are not a holiday food, potato chips on an airplane are not a vacation food. It's fine to splurge on some only-on-vacation treats or local delicacies, but do so mindfully. And make trade-offs: if you feel like dessert or wine, skip the bread and potatoes.

Remember the basics. Stick with lean protein-based meals and snacks, eat lots of vegetables, watch portion sizes, and be smart about dense carbs.

At home, get right back on track. If you can, go grocery shopping right away so you have the healthy foods you need. I also recommend having several healthful frozen options in the freezer so you don't have to order out in case you don't have time to get to the store for a day or two. Consider cycling back to the CleanStart Plan to put yourself back where you want to be.

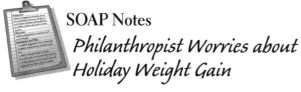

SOAP Notes
Philanthropist Worries about Holiday Weight Gain

Laura is a very busy philanthropist in her early 60s with an underactive thyroid. She was referred to me last year by her primary care doctor for weight loss and borderline high blood sugar levels. To date, she has lost 17.6 pounds (her goal was 20 pounds). This note was written one month into her program, just before the winter holiday season. She does a lot of entertaining.

Subjective:

Patient feels good, not getting hungry, but is a little frustrated at slow pace of weight loss (less than 1 pound per week). Concerned about frequent entertaining commitments over the holidays derailing her diet. Working out with a trainer for one hour, three times per week—mainly strength training with some cardio.

Objective:

Weight is unchanged from 10 days prior. Review of food journal shows excess fat consumption, including nuts and cheese on salads and coconut oil used in cooking. Eating "handfuls" of nuts as a snack. Not consistently eating lean protein at three major meals, especially lunch.

Assessment and Plan:

1. Excess fat intake: Be very careful using oil in cooking; always measure amount of coconut oil, or consider using spray oil instead. Choose either nuts or cheese on salads, not both, and measure both carefully. Estimating portions size as a "handful" is not accurate. Instead, measure out serving size and consider putting into small zip bags for the week, or buy 100-calorie packs of nuts for on-the-go snacking.

2. Inadequate lean protein: Make sure to throw lean protein on salads (not just nuts and cheese for protein, because they are higher in calories and lower in protein than chicken, fish, and other lean protein). Eat protein after strength-training workouts to build calorie-burning muscle— Greek yogurt and fruit or small protein shake are best choices.

3. Increase exercise: To offset sluggish metabolism (due to underactive thyroid, age, and low lean body mass), consider activity monitor to track and increase overall lifestyle physical activity and boost calorie burning as much as possible.

4. Entertaining/holidays: Serve (or bring) an appealing vegetable tray at all parties and dinners to facilitate guiltless snacking. Patient decided she was going to skip all desserts to stay on track, so I suggested that she "treat" herself to a Greek yogurt with a little honey after her company left.

Result:

After making the changes I suggested, Laura lost three more pounds over the holidays and became obsessed with her activity monitor—so much so that she bought one for every member of her staff for a holiday gift!

—*Melina B. Jampolis, MD*

The Power of Planning

You wouldn't go on a vacation without a plan. You wouldn't start a new business without a plan. You probably don't even go out for a night on the town without one. But when it comes to eating, you may need to brush up on your planning skills.

It is amazing to me how many people who are trying to lose weight find themselves in eating situations without a plan—and, as a result, they end up overeating or consuming foods they were trying to avoid. Having an eating plan doesn't guarantee that you'll succeed at weight loss, but it sure does increase your chances of getting to where you want to be.

You don't have to figure everything out beforehand—I'm not suggesting you plan every meal and snack a week in advance. Some people do fine with that type of planning, but most don't do well with such a rigid approach. What I mean by having a plan is to think about your eating and exercise options ahead of time. This means not only planning for healthy eating, but also for indulgences. If you have a plan, you're less likely to have your diet derailed.

For example:

- If your job keeps you on the road most of the time, be prepared. Have fruit, nuts, or protein bars handy in the car at all times. If you travel a regular route, get to know where the healthier fast-food restaurant options are.

- If you know you are going to a big dinner party or work dinner, try to eat fewer starchy carbohydrates and fats during the day to give yourself a little flexibility at dinner.

- If you are going to a holiday bash, decide in advance if you are going to have a little dessert or maybe an extra glass of wine instead. Or maybe your friend makes the best bread this side of the Mississippi, and you know you can't resist a slice or two. Plan that into your day by skipping the sandwich at lunch and having a salad with chicken instead.

- If you are going to a conference, assume that the food options may not be the most favorable. Try to start with a healthy breakfast, and have a wholesome snack on hand when the afternoon "cookie break" comes around. Believe it or not, they always have cookie breaks at medical meetings—I know, it's crazy—so I always make sure I have a protein bar with me to satisfy my sweet tooth and keep my energy level up.

It is also critical to plan to shop at least one day a week to make sure you have lots of healthy food options available at home and at the office, if necessary. The key is to not just let your meals "happen" but to have some type of plan for almost any eating situation in which you may find yourself. This can be done with very little effort utilizing the meal ideas, dining-out guide, and recipes provided later on in this book. The small amount of time you spend planning will translate into big results in weight loss and maintenance.

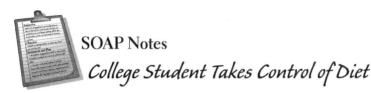

SOAP Notes
College Student Takes Control of Diet

William is a 22-year-old college student referred to me by his internist for weight loss. He was very frustrated by the fact that he had cut fast food almost completely from his diet and went to the gym three times a week, but had not lost a pound in six months. Rather than give him comprehensive instructions, I decided to keep his plan as simple as possible. He didn't want to cut bread because a sandwich was a fast and easy lunch, but he agreed to cut pasta, white potatoes, and rice as much as possible. This note includes my recommendations from our initial consultation.

Subjective:

Patient started to gain weight in high school and continued to gain gradually during college. He hates breakfast (usually skips or has a bagel) and eats out most meals because he doesn't like to cook and doesn't have a full kitchen setup. His gym workouts, which he has been doing for six months, include one hour of weight lifting and one hour of cardio three days a week. Typical eating day: no breakfast; sandwich for lunch (turkey, cheese, mayo) or pesto chicken; Chinese or Mexican takeout for dinner; limited vegetable intake; snacks consist of fruit and flavored yogurt. Drinks soda a few times a week and consumes maybe 32 ounces of water a day, with an extra 16 ounces on gym days. Reports a longtime history of snoring and occasional unpleasant gastrointestinal symptoms, but has no major medical problems.

Objective:

Height 5 feet 11 inches; weight 250 pounds; body fat 34.1%; blood pressure slightly elevated. Remainder of physical exam was normal.

Assessment and Plan:

1. Basic nutrition: Made some simple suggestions to improve his diet. Suggested having protein bar for breakfast, leaving cheese off sandwich at lunch, skipping pesto on chicken because it is high in fat, switching to whole-grain bread whenever possible, limiting takeout dinners to three times a week, limiting red meat to once a week, adding vegetables whenever possible (salad at lunch, cooked vegetables at dinner topped with Parmesan), cutting out soda, and increasing water intake to 64 ounces per day.

2. Exercise: Try interval training to boost calorie burning during workouts.

3. Sleep: Recommended patient participate in a sleep study to assess snoring—could be sleep apnea, which when untreated can make weight loss much more challenging.

Result:

William lost 45 pounds during the following seven months. He looks and feels terrific. He never had a sleep study due to insurance issues, but he reported that his snoring markedly improved with weight loss. I wasn't surprised to hear this, because weight loss is generally the first-line treatment recommendation for patients with sleep apnea.

—*Melina B. Jampolis, MD*

Coming Up Next

The next chapter is the most exciting, because it's about maintaining your hard-fought weight loss. Shedding pounds and meeting your weight-loss goal is the first step; maintaining it over time is your goal for the rest of your life. Gaining back lost weight occurs in many people, but you can beat the odds. By continuing the great habits you've learned in the pages of this book and planning ways to continue incorporating flexibility into your eating plan, you can maintain your goal weight well into the future.

CHAPTER 10

—ⱳ—

Maintaining Your Weight Loss: Seven Steps to Lifelong Success

Reaching your goal weight is an exciting milestone. All of your efforts have finally paid off, and you're probably feeling pretty fantastic. If you're like most of my successful patients, your clothing fits better (or better yet, you had to get new, smaller clothing), you're more physically fit, you feel more energetic, you are more enthusiastic about everyday life, and you are probably seeing improved results when your doctor measures things like your blood pressure, blood sugar, and cholesterol levels. If you haven't had those checked yet, I encourage you to do so.

Even though you have achieved an amazing goal, however, your journey is not over. Now it's time to start a journey of a different kind: the quest to maintain a healthy weight for the rest of your life. Here is something I always explain to my patients who achieve their goal weight: "If you go back to your old ways, you will go back to your old weight." Throughout the Doctor on Demand Diet, you've learned many habits that can serve you well for the rest of your life. Your next goal is to continue to incorporate those habits into your life permanently.

Don't let this shift intimidate you—maintaining weight loss is somewhat easier than losing, because you don't have to be quite as disciplined as before. But this next phase is not without its challenges.

Unfortunately, many of the people who lose weight regain some or all of it over the long term, most within the first year or two. This happens for a number of reasons, some that are under their control and some that are not. The trick is to do your best to manage those factors that are within your control.

201

When you lose weight, several physiological changes take place that may predispose you to regain it, including changes in your metabolism and appetite. But the good news is that you can take some important steps to counteract and minimize these changes. By continuing to make smart choices about your diet, exercise, and behavior, you can stay in charge.

In this chapter, I share with you my seven steps to lifelong weight-loss success. These steps, which are based on the proven strategies that have brought you your exciting achievement, will allow you to maintain your hard-earned weight loss for a long time to come.

Maintenance Step 1: Don't Be "Dense"

The concept of calorie density, also known as energy density, is still very important during weight-loss maintenance, because it allows you to eat larger portions while consuming fewer calories. In fact, paying attention to calorie density is especially important for weight maintenance, as my patients typically focus less on portion sizes after they reach their goal weight.

We discussed calorie density earlier, because eating low-density foods helps with weight loss. Research shows it can be a powerful tool for weight maintenance as well.

Remember, calorie density is basically the amount of calories in a given volume of food. For example, a cup of romaine lettuce has low calorie density because it is very high in water and contains fiber, while a cup of butter has a high calorie density because it is very high in fat and low in water and fiber. Your goal is to fill your plate with low-density foods, because they do the best job of filling up your stomach while keeping calorie counts low. Using calorie density to your advantage is one of the absolute keys to long-term weight loss.

Research shows that people tend to like to eat roughly the same *amount* of food most days, and that holds true whether the food they eat is lower or higher in energy density. So the density of your food really does make a difference. When you focus on choosing low-density foods, you can eat a larger amount of food with a smaller amount of calories compared with high-density foods. Eating low-density foods helps you feel fuller, less hungry, and more satiated.

When you're looking for low-density foods, you can count on vegetables. As you've discovered, increasing vegetable intake is a major part of the

Clinical Pearl: *Be a Veggie Sneak!*

Eating vegetables is a vital maintenance strategy, so I urge you to continue to include large amounts of them in your meals as often as possible. Sneak them into recipes, toss them into salads, stir them into soups, and blend them into smoothies wherever you can. Experiment with tasty and healthful vegetable recipes to keep things interesting, and choose seasonal produce whenever possible to optimize health and taste. Challenge yourself to try a new vegetable or cook an old vegetable in a new way at least once a week, and you will boost your eating satisfaction and weight-loss maintenance success. ◇

Doctor on Demand Diet. That's because they're high in fiber and water, low in calories, and low in calorie density. They're also a fantastic source of vitamins, minerals, antioxidants, and other disease-fighting nutrients. One of the most frequent mistakes that I see my patients make after they reach their goal weight and set out to maintain weight loss is slacking off on eating vegetables. This often contributes to their regaining lost weight.

 ### Research on Demand: Follow the Loser

Research on the habits of "weight-loss maintainers"— people who have lost significant amounts of weight and kept it off for a long time—can tell us a lot. A study published in 2011 in the journal *Eating Behaviors* compared the eating habits of normal-weight adults, overweight adults, and weight-loss maintainers who had lost at least 10 percent of their body weight and had kept it off for at least five years. The study found that maintainers ate more whole grains and vegetables, more fiber, and fewer calories from fat than the normal-weight or overweight subjects. And although maintainers consumed more food by weight than the other groups, they took in fewer calories, because they filled up on foods such as vegetables that have low calorie density.

The bottom line: Continuing to consume high-fiber, low energy-density foods can help you maintain your weight loss.

Maintenance Step 2: Stick with the Fundamentals

When you hit your weight-loss goal, it's tempting to ditch the fundamental dietary changes you made in order to lose weight and to slide back to your old eating habits. Don't do it! Although you can give yourself a little more wiggle room in terms of having an occasional splurge food, overall you're best served by continuing to follow the guidelines that fueled your weight loss.

Protein at breakfast is especially important, because it sets the tone for satiety and healthy eating all day. Let's face it, carbs are the easiest grab-and-go option, but making sure to start your day with protein, and continuing to consume moderate amounts of protein throughout the day, can help control the hunger that may start creeping in as your body tries to return to its old habits. Protein is also important for maintaining all that calorie-burning muscle mass that you (I hope) have worked so hard to build.

And don't get careless with fat. Fat calories can add up quickly, especially if you start eating out more often. Try to continue to limit restaurant visits to some extent, and if you do eat out often, plan ways to balance any excess fat intake with lower-fat choices the rest of the day.

As for carbohydrates, continue to pay attention to carbohydrate quality, focusing on high-fiber carbohydrates and limiting sugar and refined, highly processed carbs. Sugar-sweetened beverages are especially problematic, and research shows that limiting them as much as possible can help you stay trim.

Maintenance Step 3: Keep Cycling

When you're thinking of a weight-loss plan as a short-term commitment, it's easier to say no to high-calorie treats at restaurants or parties. But when you're making a long-term commitment to maintaining weight loss, you've got to find a way to fit in special occasions without constantly depriving yourself. Let's face it, eating is a major part of many people's social life. Restaurant meals, dinner parties, holidays, brunches, vacations, and happy hours are going to happen, and it's not always easy—or necessary—to strictly control your calories every single day.

For this reason, I often recommend that my patients consider incorporating cycling on a long-term basis, especially if they have active social lives

Secrets of Success

Much of the research on ongoing weight-loss maintenance comes from the National Weight Control Registry (NWCR), a research effort that studies and evaluates the choices and behaviors of people who have successfully lost weight and kept it off long-term. Registry members have lost an average of 66 pounds and have maintained their weight loss for an average of 5.5 years. Although NWCR members use different strategies, most follow a low-calorie, low-fat diet and do high levels of activity. For example:

- 78 percent eat breakfast every day
- 75 percent weigh themselves at least once a week
- 62 percent watch less than 10 hours of TV per week
- 90 percent exercise, on average, about an hour per day

To join or learn more about the NWCR, visit the group's website: www.nwcr.ws.

or eat out often. Eating "clean" with a cycling day even once a week can help offset the slow weight gain that many people experience while trying to maintain.

There are several ways to Diet-Cycle—you can review them by going back and rereading Phase 3: Cycle for Success. You may opt to Diet-Cycle by following the Phase 1 CleanStart Plan once a week (or more). Or you can simply cut (or cut back on) dense carbs—some of my patients choose to avoid or limit dense carbs such as bread and grains one or two days a week so they can enjoy more choices on weekends. Just be sure you're getting protein at most (if not all) meals and snacks, and that you're eating plenty of vegetables.

How often and when you Diet-Cycle depends on your preferences and your life. Many of my patients, like me, choose to Diet-Cycle on Mondays, because they have a bit more time on Sunday to plan for a satisfying but lower-calorie/lower-carb Monday. They like starting the week with a cycling day. If their weekend (or week) was especially indulgent, they sometimes decide to cycle two or three days a week to prevent the numbers on the scale from starting to creep up.

And remember, you always have the option of going back to the CleanStart Plan for a week or two. If you catch any weight gain early, you should be able to get back on track fast.

SOAP Notes
Entertaining Lawyer Craves Carbs

George is a lawyer in his 40s with insulin resistance, high cholesterol, and high blood sugar who has to do a lot of entertaining as part of his job. Here is a note written about one month into his program.

Subjective:

Patient feels good and is not eating bread, but is craving carbs at night. So he started eating a bowl of cereal before bed. Patient is also having trouble limiting wine because he entertains for work up to five nights a week. He is still not working out regularly but does walk the dog (small dog, so slow stop-and-go pace) 10 to 15 minutes, twice a day.

Objective:

Patient's weight up 0.4 pounds this week; food journal regularly shows inadequate intake of dense carbs during the day and overconsumption of wine almost every night.

Assessment and Plan:

1. Carbohydrate cravings: Inadequate daytime carbs are leading to carb cravings in the evening. Limit low-carb days to twice a week and add in one dense carb or fruit at breakfast and lunch. Consider Greek yogurt with a teaspoon of honey as late-night snack instead of cereal. When not consuming alcohol, OK to consume one cup of whole-wheat pasta at dinner twice a week.

2. Overconsumption of wine: On days that wine consumption is greater than one glass, cut out one dense carb and one or two fats to balance out extra calories. Make sure to alternate a glass of water with each glass of wine to slow down drinking pace.

3. Inadequate exercise: Discussed the possibility of walking to work twice a week, which involves more vigorous and sustained exertion; patient agreed to do his best.

Result:

The following week, George lost two more pounds and mostly stayed on track for the next few months. Eventually, he lost 30 pounds in six months and six inches off his waist.

—*Melina B. Jampolis, MD*

Maintenance Step 4: Weigh Yourself Regularly

One of the key findings of the National Weight Control Registry, as well as countless other weight-maintenance studies, is the importance of self-monitoring, and the best way to do this is to weigh yourself regularly. I recommend weighing yourself with this frequency:

- Once a week during months one, two, and three of maintenance.
- Once every two weeks for months four, five, and six of maintenance.
- Once a month thereafter, except for high-risk times (vacation, holidays, and times when you know you struggle).
- Vacation: Weigh yourself before the vacation and three days after (airplane travel can cause you to retain water, so it's better to wait a few days to allow your body time to get back to normal).
- Holidays (Halloween/Thanksgiving to New Year's Day): Weigh yourself once a week—I know it's not fun, but neither is getting on the scale January 1 and realizing you've gained 10 pounds!

In addition to weighing yourself, you need a plan of action for what to do with your results. The chart below shows my suggestions, but feel free to come up with your own. Just be sure to take action *before* things get too out of control.

Note: If your weight is higher than usual without an obvious cause, I always recommend reweighing yourself in a couple of days. Factors such as salty food, air travel, monthly hormonal fluctuation (in women), constipation, and even a challenging workout can cause a temporary increase in scale weight, which is often just water weight that does not need to be addressed.

Weight Gain	Action Step
1–2 pounds	Start tracking food intake again and reweigh yourself in 1–2 days; if your weight is still increased, add 1–2 days of cycling per week until you get back to goal.
3–5 pounds	Start tracking food intake and go back to Phase 2 of the Doctor on Demand Diet for 10 days and continue on to Phase 3 until you get back to your goal weight. If you aren't clear what caused the weight gain, spend some time reflecting on your eating over the past month. If you are aware of what caused the weight gain, think about and make note of what you could have done differently.
Greater than 5 pounds	Start tracking food intake and go back to the Phase 1 CleanStart Plan for 10 days and continue to Phase 2 or Phase 3 until you are back at your goal weight.
	If you aren't clear what caused the weight gain, spend some time reflecting on your eating over the past month. If you are aware of what caused the weight gain, think about and make note of what you could have done differently.
	Continue using a journal to track food and exercise until you are back in control.
	If you think you've been getting lax about portion sizes, start measuring your food again—especially fats (nuts, seeds, oil), dense carbs, alcohol, and any treats you may allow yourself.

Maintenance Step 5: Keep on Moving

We know exercise plays an important role in successful weight loss, but it may be even more crucial for long-term weight maintenance. Data from the NWCR finds that 90 percent of successful long-term losers exercise at least an hour a day. This may seem like more than you can handle, but in my experience, this can include not only formal exercise but also being more active in general.

And remember, if you don't have time for an hour per day during the week, try to find time to build more activity into your weekends. Whenever I go walking with a friend, I'm amazed at how many miles we cover just catching up with what's happened in our lives since the last time we got together. Or, break up your exercise into smaller increments, adding a few minutes here and a few minutes there. If you can't manage to fit in this much exercise, please don't bypass exercise altogether—you just may have to be a little more careful with your diet.

If you've let exercise slide, or if you haven't managed to make fitness part of your daily life, I advise you to go back and reread the chapter on exercise. I'm convinced there is an exercise strategy for everyone, no matter how busy you are. Finding it is just a matter of evaluating your exercise style and your schedule to determine the approach that works best for you.

Maintenance Step 6: Monitor Your Mood

We talked earlier in the book about the importance of having your head in the right place while you're working toward achieving your weight-loss goals. The same is true during maintenance. If you are anxious, stressed, or depressed, or if you are experiencing disordered eating that you have not yet addressed or that may be new, I encourage you to address these issues as soon as possible. Untreated psychological challenges can lead to poor food choices, exercise apathy, and rapid weight regain. Research shows a strong association between stress, mental disorders, and weight gain, often in people who are overweight to begin with.

If you're feeling like your emotional health is on shaky ground, go back to chapter 7 and use the assessment tools to get a handle on what problems might be affecting you. Review the helpful coping strategies, and if at any time you feel that you need some extra help, get in touch with your primary care doctor or other health-care professional.

Maintenance Step 7: Practice Flexible Restraint

Flexible restraint is a strategy that will serve you well as you work to maintain your weight loss. It's important when you're trying to shed pounds, but it's even more essential during maintenance. Essentially, practicing flexible restraint means being flexible rather than rigid about your daily eating choices.

Being flexible doesn't mean you can eat what you want. But it does mean allowing yourself some flexibility as you navigate the foods that tempt you.

Clinical Pearl: *Steer Your Boat*

There's an old saying I like: you can't control the ocean, but you can steer your own boat. In other words, you can't control many of the situations that go on around you, but you can control how you choose to respond to them. When something goes wrong, try to stop yourself and make a choice about how you will respond rather than automatically reacting in the most negative way. When you're stuck in traffic, for example, you can get upset and swear at the other drivers, or you can turn on your favorite music and enjoy having time to listen to it. I use this technique often, as there are several very stressful situations in my life that I simply can't control, and I spend a little time on a regular basis working on controlling my response to those situations rather than flying off the handle about them. It isn't easy, but with practice I'm getting better and better at it.

I'm 100 percent sure that you are not going to be able to avoid every single tempting food or beverage for the rest of your life. Research shows that the ability to practice flexible restraint—having some flexibility in your food intake, rather than rigidly avoiding all tempting foods—is one of the most important habits of people who successfully maintain weight loss.

Confidently consuming controlled portions of the foods you love may seem intimidating at first, but I can tell you from seeing thousands of patients over the past 14 years that when people are able to successfully navigate challenging eating situations, indulge on occasion in moderation, and get right back on track, their chances of long-term success are very good.

On the other hand, when patients insist on completely avoiding all the foods they love, I know that this sort of all-or-nothing mentality will not last and they will eventually give in to temptation, often overdo it, and find it difficult to get back on track.

Moving Forward

With these seven maintenance steps in mind—and with everything you've learned in the Doctor on Demand Diet—I hope that you feel confident and ready to move forward.

Food Rules Rule

One of the keys to successfully incorporating flexible restraint is to anticipate tempting eating situations, plan indulgences ahead of time as much as possible, and have a set of food rules in place that you abide by most of the time. For example:

- If you are going out for pizza, always have a salad (with light dressing and limited high-fat toppings) or vegetable/broth-based soup first, and limit yourself to one or two slices.
- If you are going out for cocktails, eat a healthy snack before you go so you aren't famished and tempted to devour an entire bowl of nuts or pretzels.
- If you are going out for ice cream, get the child-size portion or split a bowl with two scoops with a friend.
- If an unplanned indulgence comes up (like a hot-out-of-the-oven chocolate chip cookie), try to consume half a serving instead of the whole serving, and cut calories later in the day.
- If you are on vacation, choose one or two indulgences daily instead of ditching your healthy eating altogether. And sneak in physical activity as much as possible.

Flexible restraint is not about constantly challenging yourself with temptation (so don't stock the pantry or freezer with treats) but rather about indulging on occasion without guilt to avoid feelings of deprivation. Mastering this skill, which may take some time and trial and error, will go a long way toward helping you maintain the healthy weight you worked so hard to achieve.

My final piece of advice is that you never stop paying attention and always remain flexible in your approach to weight loss and weight maintenance. Just as there is no single best way to lose weight, there isn't just one best way for you to maintain your weight loss. And, as my patients discover as the years go by, what works today may not work quite as well in a few years. Long-term success requires you to continuously adapt your diet, exercise, and behavior choices to the realities of *your* life.

As time goes on, those realities will change. If you're the mother of preschoolers today, your everyday life will be quite different when those children are in middle school and high school. If you're a busy executive, your diet and exercise challenges will change after you retire from your job. If you're right smack in the middle of the mood swings of perimenopause, you can look forward to some stability when menopause finally arrives. And if you're like most people, at some point you will experience health issues—anything from a sprained ankle to a cancer diagnosis—that will require you to recalculate your approach. That's normal. Life throws lots of curve balls at us, and the best approach is to accept that unpredictability and to be prepared to make changes to accommodate it.

When new challenges arise, go back to basics and remember what worked best for you. Keeping an open mind will help you negotiate new situations in a successful way.

As you continue on your healthy-weight journey, I encourage you to always reach out for help if you need it. If friends and family can't give you what you are looking for, ask for guidance and advice from your primary care doctor, psychologists, registered dietitians, nutritionists, or other health-care professionals.

What matters most for your long-term health is getting the right care and support when you need it. Trust me, as a weight-loss physician, I know that successful long-term weight loss is not easy—but the physical and emotional payoff is huge. Believe in your ability to commit to your health and to succeed at making successful changes. And please share your success stories and tips with me by visiting my Facebook page, www.facebook.com/drmelina. Since I can't meet most of you in person, it's the next best thing.

Doctor on Demand
Sample Menus

In all phases of the Doctor on Demand Diet, you can design your daily menus to suit your own tastes and preferences. Or if you'd like, you can follow my sample plan, which is given here. Before you begin, here are a few reminders:

- These menus are designed to give you ideas and as many options as possible. All this variety is unrealistic for most people, though, and I don't expect you to have a different breakfast, lunch, and dinner every day. Feel free to choose a few favorites and repeat them throughout the week to make things simpler, and remember, you always have the option of having dinner leftovers for lunch the next day.

- Since most people don't have the time (or interest) to spend countless hours cooking, I've provided low-cook and no-cook options in the menu (with recipes in the recipe section) along with quick-fix ideas to reduce cooking time.

- Snack 1 is best consumed midafternoon. Snack 2 can be eaten as dessert after dinner or as a midmorning snack if you get hungry. It's your choice.

- If, like me, you don't enjoy the taste of plain, nonfat Greek yogurt, you can always add any of the following: one packet no-calorie sweetener, 1/4 teaspoon vanilla or almond extract, or 1/4 teaspoon cinnamon. In Phase 2 and 3 you can use low-sugar flavored yogurts if you can find them, or add a teaspoon of sugar or honey.

    ❧ Feel free to start any meal with a cup of the **Dr. Melina's Doctor on Demand (DOD) Pureed Vegetable Soup** (or store-bought; aim for broth-based soup with under 100 calories per serving) or a small green salad with one tablespoon of low-fat dressing. I recommend making a big pot of the soup each week to use as needed throughout the week.

    ❧ To make your life easier, I also recommend making recipes over the weekend that are easy to reheat and eat during the week, such as egg white cupcakes, **Dr. Melina's Power Muffins** (Phase 2), **Chipotle and Turkey Chili**, and any of my soups.

    ❧ Since I recommend *up to* two dense carbs per day in the CleanStart phase, some menus may contain less, and whole-grain sides are often optional.

Phase 1: CleanStart Sample Menu

Day #1:

Breakfast	**Strawberry Almond Parfait**
Lunch	**Mexicali Chicken Salad**
Dinner	**Broiled Fish and Garlic Vegetable Medley** + 1/2 cup cooked barley or brown rice (optional)
Snack 1	1 hard-boiled egg + 1 cup baby carrots + 2 tbsp. **Greek Yogurt Hummus**
Snack 2	Dessert: 1 **Baked Apple** + 2 tbsp. **Cinnamon Ricotta Dip**

Day #2:

Breakfast	**Oatmeal Cookie Smoothie**
Lunch	**Tuna Niçoise Salad** + 1 orange
Dinner	**Flank Steak** + 1 cup **Spiced Butternut Squash** + 1–2 cups arugula with 1 tbsp. **Basic Balsamic** (make extra flank steak for lunch tomorrow)
Snack 1	1 pear + 1 string cheese
Snack 2	Dessert: 6 oz. plain nonfat yogurt or 1/4 cup of **Sweet Ricotta**

Day #3:

Breakfast	1–2 **Egg White "Cupcakes"** or **Vegetable Scramble** + 1/2 grapefruit
Lunch	**Steak House Salad** (use leftover flank steak from last night's dinner)
Dinner	**Chicken Stir-Fry** + 1/2 cup brown rice (optional)
Snack 1	1/2 cup low-fat cottage cheese + 1 sliced cucumber dipped in Dijon dressing
Snack 2	Dessert: 1 cup sliced strawberries

Day #4:

Breakfast	**Power Oatmeal**
Lunch	**Deli Chef Salad**
Dinner	**Easy Italian Chicken** + 1–2 cups **Braised Chard and Vegetables** + 1/2 cup cooked barley (optional)
Snack 1	1 string cheese + 1 peach
Snack 2	Dessert: 1 **Baked Apple** + 2 tbsp. **Sweet Ricotta** (if you bake an extra apple, you can use it in your smoothie tomorrow morning) or 1/2 fresh sliced apple topped with 1/4 tsp. cinnamon

Day #5:

Breakfast	Apple Pie Smoothie
Lunch	Chopped Chicken Spinach Salad
Dinner	**Lemon Shrimp** + 1 cup **Quinoa Medley** + 1 cup steamed broccoli
Snack 1	14 baby carrots + 1/4 cup **Greek Yogurt Hummus**
Snack 2	Dessert: 6 oz. plain nonfat yogurt or 1/4 cup **Sweet Ricotta**

Day #6:

Breakfast	Blueberry Pecan Parfait
Lunch	Mediterranean Chicken Salad
Dinner	**Dr. Melina's Tasty Turkey Meat Loaf** + 1–2 cups **Charred Spicy Green Beans** + 1 cup **Dr. Melina's DOD Pureed Vegetable Soup**

| Snack 1 | 1/2 cup low-fat cottage cheese + 1 cup cherry tomatoes |
| Snack 2 | Dessert: 1 fresh or baked pear + 2 tbsp. **Cinnamon Ricotta Dip** (optional) |

Day #7:

Breakfast	**Pizza Scramble** + 1/2 cup berries
Lunch	Leftover **Turkey Meat Loaf** + 1–2 cups **DOD Vegetable Soup**
Dinner	**Italian-Style Tilapia** + 2 cups roasted or steamed broccoli topped with 2 tbsp. Parmesan + 1/2 cup brown rice (optional)
Snack 1	6 oz. plain nonfat yogurt + 1/2 cup berries
Snack 2	Dessert: 1 orange

Day #8:

Breakfast	**Super Antioxidant Smoothie**
Lunch	**Southwest Salmon Cobb Salad**
Dinner	**Rosemary Chicken + Zucchini Parmesan** + 1 cup **Minestrone Soup**
Snack 1	1 hard-boiled egg + 1 cup baby carrots + 2 tbsp. **Greek Yogurt Hummus**
Snack 2	Dessert: 4 oz. plain nonfat Greek yogurt mixed with 1/4 cup applesauce or 1/2 sliced apple topped with 1/4 tsp. cinnamon

Day #9:

Breakfast	**Power Oatmeal**
Lunch	**Mediterranean Tuna Salad** or leftover **Rosemary Chicken** + 1 cup **Minestrone Soup**
Dinner	**Asian Lettuce Wraps** with chicken (make extra for tasty lunch salad tomorrow) + 1 cup steamed snow peas and carrots (drizzle vegetables with the sauce from the wraps)
Snack 1	6 oz. nonfat plain Greek yogurt + 1 orange
Snack 2	Dessert: 1 cup fresh berries

Day #10

Breakfast	Overnight Applesauce Oatmeal Parfait
Lunch	Asian chicken salad (using last night's leftover) or **Mexicali Chicken Salad**
Dinner	Vegetarian Stir-Fry + 1/2 cup brown rice (optional)
Snack 1	Snack-size **Oatmeal Cookie Smoothie**
Snack 2	Dessert: 1 **Baked Pear** (or 1 fresh pear) + 2 tbsp. **Sweet Ricotta** (optional)

Phase 2: Customize Your Carbs Sample Menu

This menu is designed as a basic meal plan for Phase 2 INSULIN-RESISTANT dieters, although this type of diet can work for both groups. If you are insulin responsive and prefer more carbs, it can easily be modified by cutting back on fat at any meal or snack and adding a full or half serving of dense carb or fruit instead.

Day #1

Breakfast	**Dr. Melina's Power Muffin** + 6 oz. low-sugar Greek yogurt
Lunch	**Crunchy Gazpacho-Style Salad** with shrimp
Dinner	**Beef Flank Stir-Fry** + 1/2 cup brown rice (optional)
Snack 1	1 orange + 2 tbsp. almonds (or 100 calorie pack)
Snack 2	Dessert: **Baked Apple** with cinnamon topped with 2 tbsp. **Honey Ricotta Crunch**

Day #2

Breakfast	Piña Colada Smoothie
Lunch	**Grilled Chicken TBLT Wrap**
Dinner	Fish Tacos + side salad + 2 tbsp. **Southwest Vinaigrette**
Snack 1	14 baby carrots + 1/4 cup **Green Goddess-Style Yogurt Dip**
Snack 2	Dessert: 4 oz. low-sugar yogurt + 1 tbsp. sunflower seeds

Day #3

Breakfast	Vegetable Scramble Breakfast Burrito
Lunch	Gourmet Arugula Chicken Salad
Dinner	Vegetarian Lasagna Rolls + 1–2 cups **Dr. Melina's DOD Pureed Vegetable Soup**
Snack 1	1 apple + 1 tbsp. peanut butter
Snack 2	Dessert: 1/4 cup **Sweet Ricotta** with 1/2 cup sliced strawberries

Day #4

Breakfast	Power Oatmeal
Lunch	Deli Chef Salad Pita Pocket + 1 apple
Dinner	Flank Steak with Chimichurri Sauce + Creamed Spinach + 1/2 cup steamed or **Roasted Carrots**
Snack 1	1/2 cup low-fat cottage cheese + 1/2 cup pineapple
Snack 2	Dessert: 4 oz. low-sugar yogurt + 1 tbsp. chopped nuts

Day #5

Breakfast	Cashew Coconut Parfait
Lunch	Herbed Tuna Melt + 1–2 cups **Dr. Melina's DOD Pureed Vegetable Soup**
Dinner	Chipotle and Turkey Chili + 1 cup steamed broccoli + side salad + 2 tbsp. **Southwest Vinaigrette**
Snack 1	1 orange + 2 tbsp. almonds (or 100 calorie pack)
Snack 2	Dessert: 1 cup berries + 2 tbsp. whipped topping

Day #6

Breakfast	Berry Green Banana Smoothie
Lunch	Turkey Hummus Wrap or leftover **Chipotle and Turkey Chili** + 1 cup baby carrots + 2 tbsp. **Greek Yogurt Hummus**
Dinner	4 oz. grilled or baked chicken (make extra for lunch tomorrow) + **Quinoa Medley** + 1–2 cups **Roasted Cauliflower**
Snack 1	2 celery sticks + 1 tbsp. peanut butter
Snack 2	Dessert: 1/2 sliced banana + 4 oz. yogurt

Day #7

Breakfast	Easy Breakfast Sandwich + 1/2 grapefruit
Lunch	Mexicali Chicken Salad
Dinner	Shrimp Stir-Fry + 1/2 cup brown rice (optional)
Snack 1	1 pear + 1 string cheese
Snack 2	Dessert: Honey Ricotta Crunch

Day #8

Breakfast	Banana Nut Parfait
Lunch	Mediterranean Chicken or Tuna Pita Pocket + 14 baby carrots + 1/4 cup Green Goddess-Style Yogurt Dip
Dinner	Pork "Adobo" Style + 1–2 cups Charred Spicy Green Beans + 1/2 cup cooked barley
Snack 1	Snack-size Oatmeal Cookie Smoothie
Snack 2	Dessert: 1 cup berries + 2 tbsp. whipped topping

Day #9

Breakfast	Mexican Scramble + 1 orange
Lunch	BBQ Chicken Pita Pizza + side salad with 1 tbsp. dressing
Dinner	Dr. Melina's Tasty Turkey Meat Loaf + 1–2 cups Cauliflower Mash + 1 cup Dr. Melina's DOD Pureed Vegetable Soup
Snack 1	6 oz. low-sugar yogurt + 1 tbsp. chia seeds or chopped nuts
Snack 2	Dessert: Baked Apple with cinnamon + 2 tbsp. Cinnamon Ricotta

Day #10

Breakfast	Double Chocolate Cherry Chia Smoothie
Lunch	Southwest Salmon Cobb Salad or leftover Turkey Meat Loaf + 1 cup DOD Vegetable Soup
Dinner	Sweet and Spicy Mango Chicken + 1 cup Spiced Butternut Squash + arugula side salad with 1 tbsp. Basic Vinaigrette

| Snack 1 | 1 serving whole-grain crackers + 1 slice low-fat cheese or 2 wedges spreadable cheese |
| Snack 2 | Dessert: 1 cup berries + 2 tbsp. whipped topping |

Phase 3: Cycle for Success Sample Menu

This menu is designed as a basic meal plan for Phase 3 INSULIN-RESISTANT dieters, although this type of diet can also work for the insulin-responsive dieter. It features cycling days containing no dense carbs. If you are insulin-responsive and prefer not to cut dense carbs completely on your cycling day, you can substitute No Dense Carb days with any Phase 1 CleanStart day.

Day #1 (No Dense Carbs day)

Breakfast	Super Antioxidant Smoothie
Lunch	Deli Chef Salad
Dinner	Shrimp Stir-Fry + side salad with 1–2 tbsp. **Asian Vinaigrette** or 1 cup miso soup
Snack 1	1 apple + 1 tbsp. peanut butter
Snack 2	Dessert: 1/4 cup **Cinnamon Ricotta Dip/Crunch** topped with 1 tbsp. chopped walnuts

Day #2

Breakfast	Dr. Melina's Power Muffin + 6 oz. Greek yogurt
Lunch	Southwest Chicken Cobb Salad
Dinner	Italian-Style Tilapia + 1–2 cups **Garlic Vegetable Medley** + 1/2 cup brown rice
Snack 1	1 orange + 2 tbsp. nuts (or 100 calorie pack)
Snack 2	Dessert: 1 cup berries + 1/4 cup **Sweet Ricotta**

Day #3 (No Dense Carbs day)

Breakfast	Vegetable Scramble + 1 cup cantaloupe
Lunch	Tuna Niçoise Salad
Dinner	Flank Steak + 1–2 cups **Roasted Brussels Sprouts** + 1–2 cups **Dr. Melina's DOD Pureed Vegetable Soup**

| Snack 1 | 2 tbsp. almonds (or 100 calorie pack) + 1 pear |
| Snack 2 | Dessert: 6 oz. low-sugar yogurt + 1 tbsp. chia seeds |

Day #4

Breakfast	Power Oatmeal
Lunch	Mediterranean Chicken Salad + 1 cup grapes
Dinner	Dr. Melina's Tasty Turkey Meat Loaf + 1–2 cups Cauliflower Mash + 1–2 cups Dr. Melina's DOD Pureed Vegetable Soup
Snack 1	6 oz. yogurt + 1 tbsp. chopped nuts
Snack 2	Dessert: Honey Ricotta Crunch

Day #5

Breakfast	Crunchy Pear Parfait
Lunch	Leftover Turkey Meat Loaf + 14 baby carrots + 1/4 cup Green Goddess-Style Yogurt Dip
Dinner	Rosemary Chicken + Zucchini Parmesan + 1 cup Minestrone Soup + glass of wine (Flex Block)
Snack 1	1 hard-boiled egg + 2 mandarin oranges/cuties
Snack 2	Dessert: 1/4 cup Cinnamon Ricotta Dip/Crunch topped with 1 tbsp. chopped almonds

Day #6

Breakfast	Peach Cobbler Smoothie
Lunch	Chopped Chicken Spinach Salad + small whole-grain roll or 1/2 whole-grain pita (optional)
Dinner	Beef Flank Stir-Fry + 1/2 cup brown rice + glass of wine (Flex Block)
Snack 1	6 oz. yogurt + 1 tbsp. chopped nuts
Snack 2	Dessert: Baked Apple with cinnamon + 2 tbsp. Cinnamon Ricotta Dip/Crunch

Day #7

| Breakfast | Pizza Scramble Burrito + 1/2 grapefruit |
| Lunch | Deli Chef Salad + 1 peach |

Dinner	Lemon Shrimp + 1 cup **Quinoa Medley** + 1–2 cups **Dr. Melina's DOD Pureed Vegetable Soup** + **Baked Apple Crumble** (Flex Block)
Snack 1	Protein bar
Snack 2	Dessert: 6 oz. yogurt

Day #8 (No Dense Carbs day)

Breakfast	**Strawberry Almond Parfait**
Lunch	**Crunchy Gazpacho-Style Salad** with shrimp + 1 apple
Dinner	**Easy Italian Chicken** + 2 cups **Braised Chard and Vegetables**
Snack 1	1 hard-boiled egg + 1 cup baby carrots
Snack 2	Dessert: 1/4 cup **Sweet Ricotta** topped with 1 tbsp. slivered almonds

Day #9

Breakfast	1–2 **Egg White "Cupcakes"** (sweet potato variation) + 1/2 banana
Lunch	**Grilled Chicken TBLT Wrap** + side salad with 1–2 tbsp. **Basic Vinaigrette**
Dinner	**Chipotle and Turkey Chili** + 2 cups steamed broccoli (serve Dr. Melina style and pour chili over broccoli)
Snack 1	1/2 sliced banana + 6 oz. yogurt
Snack 2	Dessert: 1 cup berries + 1/4 cup **Sweet Ricotta**

Day #10

Breakfast	**Mango Mint Smoothie**
Lunch	Leftover **Chipotle and Turkey Chili** + 14 baby carrots + 2 tbsp. **Greek Yogurt Hummus**
Dinner	**Shrimp Tacos** + side salad with 1–2 tbsp. **Southwest Vinaigrette**
Snack 1	1 sliced apple + 1 tbsp. peanut butter
Snack 2	6 oz. yogurt

Doctor on Demand Grocery Essentials

Although nearly all of the foods I recommend in the Doctor on Demand Diet are healthy staples available in your local supermarket, it can be helpful to have a list with you as you do your shopping. Use the following as a guide, but feel free to customize it to satisfy your own preferences. This is a list of the basics needed to get started on CleanStart, the first phase of the Doctor on Demand Diet. For the second phase, Customize Your Carbs, you can add bread products and a greater variety of dense carbs, protein, dairy protein, and fruit.

Pure Protein

☐ Eggs
☐ Protein powder (optional)

Lean protein

☐ Fish
☐ Poultry
☐ Shellfish
☐ Lean red meat

Dairy Protein

☐ Plain yogurt (Greek or regular)
☐ Part-skim shredded mozzarella
☐ String cheese
☐ Low-fat cottage cheese
☐ Low-fat ricotta
☐ Blue cheese crumbles
☐ Fresh grated Parmesan

Fatty Protein

☐ Nuts (whole and/or slivered)
☐ Seeds (flax, chia, and/or sunflower)

Starchy Protein

☐ Beans (dried or canned—black, kidney, garbanzo)
☐ Lentils

Dense Carbs

- ☐ Whole grains:
  - ☐ quinoa
  - ☐ barley
  - ☐ brown rice
- ☐ Sweet potatoes
- ☐ Peas
- ☐ Corn

Low-Sugar Fruit

- ☐ Berries (fresh or frozen)
- ☐ Apples
- ☐ Pears
- ☐ Grapefruit
- ☐ Oranges
- ☐ Peaches (fresh or frozen)
- ☐ Apricots

Vegetables

- ☐ Lettuce
- ☐ Broccoli (fresh or frozen)
- ☐ Carrots (fresh or frozen)
- ☐ Cauliflower (fresh or frozen)
- ☐ Kale
- ☐ Spinach (fresh or frozen)
- ☐ Green beans (fresh or frozen)
- ☐ Mushrooms
- ☐ Onions
- ☐ Peppers
- ☐ Cucumber
- ☐ Tomatoes (fresh and canned)
- ☐ Celery
- ☐ Zucchini

Healthy Fats

- ☐ Olive oil
- ☐ Canola oil
- ☐ Avocado
- ☐ Hummus

Spices/Miscellaneous

- ☐ Cinnamon
- ☐ Turmeric
- ☐ Cumin
- ☐ Chili powder
- ☐ Onion powder
- ☐ Garlic powder
- ☐ Basil
- ☐ Oregano
- ☐ Cilantro
- ☐ Parsley
- ☐ Garlic
- ☐ Ginger
- ☐ Dijon mustard
- ☐ Vinegar (apple cider, balsamic)
- ☐ Low-sodium vegetable broth
- ☐ Low-sodium soy sauce
- ☐ Salsa
- ☐ Stevia (or preferred no-calorie sweetener)
- ☐ Green tea

Doctor on Demand Recipes

- For all of the recipes, I have provided only the number of dense carbs and/or fat per serving to keep things simple. These are the most important categories to track. Protein amounts range based on your size, two servings of dairy and fruit are built into every daily menu plan, and vegetables are plentiful if you use my recipes.

- To save you time during meal preparation, I have provided QUICK FIX options whenever possible.

- You will notice that spices are plentiful in many of these recipes due to their ability to improve insulin resistance and add flavor without fat. If you use your own recipes, I strongly encourage you to add spices whenever possible.

BREAKFASTS

Build a Better Smoothie

Step 1: **Choose a protein.** Use 6 oz. plain low-fat or nonfat yogurt (Greek or Icelandic is best because it is double the protein of regular yogurt) or 1 scoop of protein powder.

Step 2: **Add 1 serving of fruit** (fresh or frozen) **or dense carb** (oats). Choose lower-sugar/higher-fiber fruits only for Phase 1 (Clean-Start).

Step 3: **Add 1 serving of healthy fat.** This helps you feel fuller longer. Choose nuts, seeds, or nut milk, which will serve as liquid for next step.

225

Choosing a Protein Powder

Some research suggests that dairy proteins, especially whey protein, may be particularly beneficial in terms of weight loss, muscle gain, improving insulin response, and hunger control. If you are vegetarian, soy protein or plant protein blends are good choices. Aim for a product with 14–21 grams of protein per serving (which is the equivalent of 2–3 ounces of pure protein) and as little added sugar as possible (aim for less than 5 grams). You don't really need any fancy vitamins and minerals added, as you are going to be adding lots of healthy, real-food nutrient sources to your diet. If you are on a budget, consider buying your protein powder online or at a big box store.

Step 4: **Add a liquid.** Use 1 cup water (or 1/2 cup if using yogurt) or unsweetened almond milk (counts as 1 fat) or unsweetened coconut beverage (the kind in a box, not in a can—counts as 1 fat).

Step 5: **Add optional ingredients.** Toss in a handful of greens to boost nutrition, or add spices, extracts, or no-calorie sweeteners to boost flavor.

Step 6: **Add ice to desired consistency.** Blend until smooth.*

*For a snack-size smoothie, cut the recipe in half or skip the fat and stick with water as your liquid choice.

Note: These are guidelines, not rules. Feel free to make modifications to fit your meal preferences. For example, if you prefer to skip the fat in step 3 and save it for another meal, go right ahead. If you don't want to waste a dense carb on a smoothie, stick with only fruit. This is your plan, so do what works best for you.

Phases 2 & 3 modifications:

- Expand fruit options to include all fruits.
- For your liquid, you can choose 1 cup fat-free or plain soy milk + 1/2 scoop of protein powder or 3 oz. yogurt.
- Insulin-resistant: May add additional serving of healthy fat.
- Insulin-responsive: May use 1 serving of fruit + 1/2 to 1 serving of dense carbs.

Oatmeal Cookie Smoothie   (all phases ♦ 1 fat, 1 dense carb)
1 serving

Vanilla protein powder	1 scoop
Rolled oats, uncooked	1/4 cup
Unsweetened vanilla almond milk	1 cup
Vanilla extract	1 tsp.
Cinnamon	1/4 tsp.
Nutmeg	1/8 tsp.
Ice	to desired consistency

Combine ingredients in a blender and blend until smooth.

Apple Pie Smoothie   (all phases ♦ 1 fat) 1 serving

Apple, cored and sliced	1
or	
Unsweetened applesauce	1/2 cup
Apple pie spice*	1 tsp.
Plain nonfat Greek yogurt	6 oz.
or	
Vanilla protein powder	1 scoop
Ground flaxseed	1 heaping tbsp.
Water	1/2 to 1 cup
Ice	to desired consistency

*If you don't have apple pie spice, use 1/4 tsp. cinnamon, 1/8 tsp. nutmeg, and a dash of allspice.

Combine ingredients in a blender and blend until smooth.

Super Antioxidant Smoothie   (all phases ♦ 1 fat)
1 serving

Vanilla protein powder	1 scoop
Blueberries, fresh or frozen	1 cup
Spinach or baby kale, fresh	1 large handful
Ground flaxseed	1 heaping tbsp.
Green tea, cold	1 cup
Lemon juice	2 tsp.
Stevia (optional)	1 packet

Combine ingredients in a blender and blend until smooth.

Clinical Pearl: *Love the Lemon*

Adding lemon juice to green tea helps release its powerful antioxidants. Be sure to stir some in to your next cup. ◇

Peach Cobbler Smoothie　　(Phases 2 & 3 ◆ 1 fat, 1/2 dense carb)
1 serving

Peach, cut in quarters*	1
Ginger, grated	1 tsp. or 1/4 tsp. ginger powder
Vanilla extract	1 tsp.
Plain or vanilla protein powder	1 scoop
Rolled oats, uncooked	2 tbsp.
Ground flaxseed	1 heaping tbsp.
Cinnamon	1 dash or 1/8 tsp.
Water	1/2 cup
Ice	to desired consistency

*If peaches are out of season or unavailable in your area, use 1 cup of frozen peaches.

Combine ingredients in a blender and blend until smooth.

Berry Green Banana Smoothie　　(Phases 2 & 3 ◆ 1 fat)
1 serving

Banana	1/2 medium
Strawberries, fresh or frozen	1/2 cup
Spinach, fresh	1 large handful
Vanilla protein powder	1/2 scoop
Unsweetened coconut milk beverage	1 cup
Ice	1 cup

Combine ingredients in a blender and blend until smooth.

Double Chocolate Cherry Chia Smoothie　　(Phases 2 & 3 ◆ 1 fat)
1 serving

Chocolate protein powder	1 scoop
Frozen cherries	3/4 cup
Unsweetened cocoa powder	1 heaping tbsp.

Chia seed	1 tbsp.
Water	1 cup
Ice	to desired consistency
Stevia (optional)	1 packet

Combine ingredients in a blender and blend until smooth.

Piña Colada Smoothie
(Phases 2 & 3 ♦ 2 fats)
1 serving

Vanilla protein powder	1 scoop
Unsweetened coconut milk beverage	1 cup
Pineapple, fresh or frozen	1/2 cup
Shredded coconut	1 heaping tbsp.
Ice	to desired consistency

Combine ingredients in a blender and blend until smooth.

Mango Mint Smoothie
(Phases 2 & 3 ♦ 1 fat)
1 serving

Unsweetened vanilla almond milk	1 cup
Mango, fresh or frozen	1 cup
Ginger, grated	1 tsp. or 1/2 inch piece chopped
Mint, rough chopped	1 sprig
Plain nonfat Greek yogurt	6 oz.

Combine ingredients in a blender and blend until smooth. If you are using fresh mango, add ice to taste.

Build a Better Breakfast Parfait

Step 1: **Start with yogurt.** Use 6 oz. plain nonfat or low-fat yogurt (Greek or Icelandic is best because it is double the protein of regular yogurt).

Step 2: **Add fruit or dense carb.** Add 1 serving of fruit or dense carb or 1/2 fruit serving + 1/2 dense carb (oats or granola).

Step 3: **Add 1 serving of healthy fat.**

Step 4: **Combine.** In a breakfast-sized bowl, combine yogurt with optional add-ins (spices, extracts, and no-calorie sweetener) and top with fruit, fat, and/or dense carbs and serve.

Phases 2 & 3 modifications:

- ☙ Expand fruit options to include all fruit.
- ☙ You may use flavored yogurts (no fruit at the bottom) but aim for 12 grams or less of sugar or add 1 tsp. sugar or honey.
- ☙ Insulin-resistant: May add additional serving of healthy fat.
- ☙ Insulin-responsive: May add additional 1/2 serving of dense carb.

Strawberry Almond Parfait   (all phases ♦ 1 fat)
                                             1 serving

Plain nonfat Greek yogurt	6 oz.
Strawberries, sliced	1 cup
Almonds, sliced or chopped*	1 tbsp.
Almond extract (optional)	1/2 tsp.
Stevia (optional)	1 packet

*I like chopped almonds best so I get whole roasted almonds, put 7 in a plastic bag, and crush them up.

In a breakfast-sized bowl, combine yogurt with almond extract and stevia and top with strawberries and almonds.

Blueberry Pecan Parfait   (all phases ♦ 1 fat)
                                             1 serving

Plain nonfat Greek yogurt	6 oz.
Cinnamon	1/8 tsp.
Blueberries	3/4 cup
Pecans, chopped	1 tbsp.
Stevia (optional)	1 packet
Pure maple syrup (Phases 2 and 3 only)	2 tsp.

In a breakfast-sized bowl, combine yogurt with cinnamon and stevia and top with blueberries and pecans.

OPTION: I also enjoy this with 1 tbsp. of chia seeds mixed into the yogurt instead of the pecans for an extra boost of super-satisfying soluble fiber.

Clinical Pearl: Chow on Chia

Because of the soluble fiber in chia seeds, they form a gel within a few minutes when combined with the liquid in the yogurt, which can help keep you fuller longer. To optimize this hunger-busting effect, let yogurt and chia mix sit for five minutes before serving. ◇

Overnight Applesauce Oatmeal Parfait

(all phases ♦ 1 fat, 1 dense carb)
1 serving

Plain nonfat Greek yogurt	6 oz.
Unsweetened applesauce	1/4 cup
Rolled oats, uncooked	1/4 cup
Cinnamon	1/4 tsp.
Almonds, chopped	1 tbsp.
Stevia (optional)	1 packet

Combine all ingredients except almonds, mix well, and refrigerate overnight. Before serving in a breakfast-sized bowl, top with 1 tbsp. chopped almonds.

QUICK FIX: If you don't have time to make ahead, use 1/4 cup reduced-fat granola or 1/2 cup high-fiber cereal (aim for 3–5 grams of fiber per serving) instead of rolled oats. Combine the yogurt, applesauce, cinnamon, and stevia and top with granola or cereal and almonds.

Crunchy Pear Parfait

(Phases 2 & 3 ♦ 1 fat, 1/2 dense carb)
1 serving

Pear, chopped	1/2
Plain nonfat Greek yogurt	6 oz.
or	
Low-sugar vanilla Greek yogurt	6 oz.
Low-fat granola	2 tbsp.
Ground flaxseed	1 tbsp.
Cinnamon or nutmeg (optional)	1/8 tsp.
Stevia (optional)	1 packet

In a breakfast-sized bowl, combine yogurt with granola, flaxseed, spices, and stevia and mix well. Top with pear and serve.

Cashew Coconut Parfait (Phases 2 & 3 ♦ 1 fat, 1/2 dense carb)
                                                                1 serving

Plain nonfat Greek yogurt	6 oz.
or	
Low-sugar vanilla Greek yogurt	6 oz.
Toasted and shredded coconut	1 tbsp.
Turmeric	1/8 tsp.
Cashews, chopped	1 tbsp.
Low-fat granola	2 tbsp.
Banana, sliced (optional)	1/2

In a breakfast-sized bowl, combine yogurt with coconut and turmeric and top with cashews, granola, and banana.

Banana Nut Parfait (Phases 2 & 3 ♦ 1 fat)
                                                                1 serving

Plain nonfat Greek yogurt	6 oz.
or	
Low-sugar vanilla Greek yogurt	6 oz.
Pumpkin pie spice	1/2 tsp.
Banana, sliced	1/2
Walnuts, chopped	1 tbsp.
Stevia (optional)	1 packet

In a breakfast-sized bowl, combine the yogurt with the pumpkin pie spice and stevia and top with banana and walnuts.

Power Oatmeal (Phase 1 ♦ 1 dense carb; Phases 2 & 3 ♦ 2 dense carbs)
                                                                1 serving

Step 1: **Cook oats.** Phase 1 serving size is 1/4 cup raw (1/2 cup cooked) oats; Phase 2 and 3 serving size is 1/2 cup raw (1 cup cooked) oats.

Step 2: **Add protein.** Combine 1/2 scoop protein powder with 1/4 cup water and mix into cooked oatmeal, or eat protein on the side: 6 oz. cup plain nonfat Greek yogurt, 1 egg (hard-boiled or scrambled), or 1/2 cup nonfat cottage cheese.

Step 3: **Add 1 serving of healthy fat.**

OPTION: To boost the flavor, add your choice of spices, extracts, or no-calorie sweetener.

Phases 2 & 3 modifications:

- ✿ Insulin-responsive: May add 2 tbsp. of raisins.
- ✿ Insulin-resistant: May add additional serving of healthy fat.

Oatmeal topping options (1 fat):

- ✿ Pecan (1 tbsp.), cinnamon (1/8 tsp.), no-calorie sweetener (optional)
- ✿ Almonds, slivered (1 tbsp.), cinnamon (1/8 tsp.), ginger powder (1/8 tsp.), no-calorie sweetener (optional)
- ✿ Walnuts, chopped (1 tbsp.), pumpkin pie spice (1/4 tsp.), no-calorie sweetener (optional)

 Clinical Pearl: The Best Way to Cook Oatmeal

Slow-cooking oatmeal is best because when it's eaten after being cooked this way, it raises blood sugar the most gradually (which also leads to a more gradual drop). But it takes a long time to cook, so if you enjoy oatmeal at breakfast, consider cooking a pot over the weekend to heat and eat all week. ◇

Savory Scrambles (all phases) and Breakfast Burritos (Phases 2 & 3)

Mexican Scramble   **(1 fat, 1/2 dense carb)**
                                                      1 serving

Egg whites	2
Egg, whole	1
Black beans	1/4 cup
Avocado, sliced	1/4
Salsa or pico de gallo	1/4 cup

Bring a nonstick pan to medium heat, remove from heat, and coat lightly with nonstick cooking spray. Mix egg and egg whites in small bowl. Add egg mix to pan and cook until firm, with no liquid remaining. Add beans for 1 minute to warm and top with avocado and salsa or pico de gallo.

Vegetable Scramble (0 fat, 0 dense carbs)
1 serving

Spinach	1/2 cup
Mushrooms, sliced	1/2 cup
Yellow or Vidalia onion, diced	1/4 cup
Egg whites	2
Egg, whole	1

Bring a nonstick pan to medium-high heat, remove from heat, and coat lightly with nonstick cooking spray. Mix egg and egg whites in small bowl and set aside. Add vegetables and cook for 3–5 minutes until soft. Add eggs, reduce heat to medium, and cook until firm.

Pizza Scramble (0 fat, 0 dense carbs)
1 serving

Egg whites	3
Yellow onion, diced	1/4 cup
Red pepper, diced	1/4 cup
Marinara sauce	2 tbsp.
Mozzarella, shredded	2 heaping tbsp.

Bring a nonstick pan to medium-high heat, remove from heat, and coat lightly with nonstick cooking spray. Add onions and red peppers and cook for 3–5 minutes until soft. Add eggs, reduce heat to medium, and cook until firm. Add marinara sauce and mozzarella, cover pan with lid, turn off heat, and leave covered until cheese has melted.

OPTION: For Phases 2 and 3, all of these scrambles can be transformed into a breakfast burrito using a small whole-wheat flour tortilla or wrap (100 calories or less). Burrito style will add 1 dense carb.

Egg White "Cupcakes" (all phases)

Spinach, Broccoli, and Onion (0 fat, 0 dense carbs)
12 servings

Spinach, frozen, chopped	1 package, 16 oz.
Broccoli, fresh or frozen, chopped small	4 cups
Yellow onion, small, diced	1 cup

Garlic, chopped	1 tbsp.
Egg whites	9
Whole eggs	3
Parmesan cheese	1/4 cup + (12 tsp. to top all "cupcakes")
Kosher salt	1 tsp.
Black pepper	1/4 tsp.

Preheat oven to 375 degrees. Bring a nonstick sauté pan to medium heat, remove from heat, and coat lightly with nonstick cooking spray. Add the onions and cook until brown. Add the garlic and cook for another 3 minutes. Remove from heat and place in a medium-size bowl. Defrost the spinach and broccoli (if frozen) and squeeze out any excess water, then chop the spinach and broccoli, add to the onion mix in the bowl, and set aside. In a small bowl, combine the eggs, egg whites, Parmesan cheese, salt, and pepper. Mix well and then add to vegetable mix. Spray nonstick cupcake pan with cooking oil and fill the molds approximately 3/4 full. This will make 12 "cupcakes." Top each of the cupcakes with 1 tsp. of Parmesan. Bake in the oven for 33–38 minutes. Remove from oven, let cool, pop out of pan with a spoon, and enjoy! These can be stored in the refrigerator for 2–3 days and reheated or frozen and reheated.

Variations:

Cauliflower, Kale, and Peppers

(0 fat, 0 dense carbs)
12 servings

Cauliflower	2 cups
Kale, shredded	2 cups
Roasted red peppers*	2 cups

*If you use roasted red peppers in a jar, drain well and pat dry with paper towels.

Bring a medium nonstick sauté pan to medium-high heat, remove from heat, and coat lightly with nonstick cooking spray. Add cauliflower, cook for 5 minutes, then add the kale and peppers. Cook another minute and remove from heat. Drain any excess liquid. In a separate bowl, combine eggs, egg whites, Parmesan cheese, salt, and pepper. Once slightly cool, add vegetables to egg mix. Fill your cupcake molds with egg mix and bake at 375 degrees for 33–38 minutes.

OPTION: During the last 5 minutes of cooking, top each cupcake with 1 tbsp. of shredded part-skim mozzarella.

Swiss Chard, Leeks, and Peppers
(0 fat, 0 dense carbs)
12 servings

Swiss chard	2 cups
Leeks, chopped	2 cups
Bell pepper, diced	2 cups

Bring a medium nonstick sauté pan to medium-high heat, remove from heat, and coat lightly with nonstick cooking spray. Add Swiss chard, leeks, and peppers and cook for 5 minutes, then remove from heat. In a separate bowl, combine eggs, egg whites, Parmesan cheese, salt, and pepper. Once slightly cool, add vegetables to egg mix. Fill your cupcake molds with egg mix and bake at 375 degrees for 33–38 minutes.

OPTION: During the last 5 minutes of cooking, top each cupcake with 1 tbsp. of shredded Swiss cheese or Gruyère.

Sweet Potato, Spinach, and Onion
(0 fat, 0 dense carbs)
12 servings

Sweet potato, cooked, diced*	1 cup
Spinach, chopped	2 cups
Yellow or Vidalia onion, diced	2 cups

*Sweet potato can be baked whole for an hour in the oven at 375 degrees or microwaved for about 8 minutes until tender. Dice sweet potato after baking.

Bring a medium nonstick sauté pan to medium-high heat, remove from heat, and coat lightly with nonstick cooking spray. Add the onions and cook for 3 minutes, add the spinach and cook for another minute, add the sweet potato and cook for 3 minutes, and remove from heat. In a separate bowl, combine eggs, egg whites, Parmesan cheese, salt, and pepper. Once slightly cool, add vegetables to egg mix. Fill your cupcake molds with egg mix and bake at 375 degrees for 33–38 minutes.

OPTION: During the last 5 minutes of cooking, top each cupcake with 1 tbsp. of shredded part-skim mozzarella.

Dr. Melina's Power Muffins (Phases 2 & 3 ◆ 1½ fats, 1 dense carb)
12 servings (1 muffin per serving)

Whole-wheat flour	1 cup
Ground almond meal	1/2 cup
Ground flaxseed	1/4 cup
Baking soda	1 tsp.
Baking powder	1 tsp.
Salt	1/2 tsp.
Cinnamon	1/4 tsp.
Banana, very ripe	3 medium
Brown sugar	1/4 cup
Egg, beaten	1
Butter, melted	1/4 cup

Preheat oven to 375 degrees. Coat muffin pan lightly with nonstick cooking spray. Mix flour, almond meal, flaxseed, baking soda, baking powder, salt, and cinnamon in large bowl. Mash bananas in smaller bowl and add brown sugar, beaten egg, and melted butter. Add banana mix to dry mix and stir. Divide into muffin cups about 3/4 full and bake for 18–20 minutes.

Easy Breakfast Sandwich   (Phases 2 & 3 ◆ 1 dense carb)
1 serving

Light whole-grain English muffin*	1
Egg, whole	1
Turkey bacon or ham, cooked	1 oz.
Reduced-fat cheese	1 slice

*If you use a regular English muffin, count as 1½ dense carbs.

Toast English muffin. Coat pan lightly with nonstick cooking spray and scramble or fry egg. Top toasted English muffin with cooked egg. Top with turkey bacon or ham and slice of cheese. Heat if desired to melt cheese.

ENTRÉES

Vegetarian Stir-Fry   (all phases ◆ 1 fat)
                                                                    4 servings

For the vegetable medley:

Sesame oil	1 tbsp.
Broccoli slaw	1 bag, 10–12 oz.
Mushrooms, sliced	16 oz.
Bean sprouts	1 bag, 10–12 oz.
Edamame, shelled, or tofu, cubed*	2 cups edamame or 20 oz. tofu

For the sauce:

Soy sauce	1/4 cup + 2 tsp.
Garlic, minced	2 tsp. or 1/4 tsp. powder
Ginger, minced	2 tsp. or 1/4 tsp. powder
Scallions, chopped	1/4 cup

*If you are using tofu, cook tofu first for 8–10 minutes on medium-high heat in a nonstick pan coated lightly with nonstick cooking spray. Add 2 tbsp. of sauce, cook for additional 1–2 minutes, and set aside. Then cook vegetables as above, combine with tofu and remainder of sauce, and cook for additional 1–2 minutes.

In a small bowl, mix together the soy sauce, garlic, ginger, and scallions and set aside. Combine vegetables in a bowl and set aside. In a nonstick pan over medium-high heat, add sesame oil, then add all ingredients to pan and sauté for about 5–7 minutes, stirring frequently. Drain excess water if necessary. Pour in the sauce, cook for another minute, and remove from heat.

QUICK FIX: To save on preparation time, opt for the powdered ginger and garlic over the fresh, use two 8 oz. packages of presliced mushrooms, and buy the tofu already cubed and ready to go.

Stir-Fry Variations:

Shrimp Stir-Fry   (all phases ◆ 1 fat)
                                                                    4 servings

Shrimp	1 lb.
Mushrooms, sliced	1 container, 8–10 oz.

Yellow squash, sliced	1 large
Zucchini, sliced	1 large
Yellow or white onion, sliced	1
Snow peas	2 cups or 1 bag, 8 oz.
Bean sprouts	1 bag, 8–10 oz.
Sesame oil	1 tbsp.

Beef Flank Stir-Fry

(all phases ♦ 1 fat)
4 servings

Lean beef flank, sliced	1 lb. bite-size slices
Broccoli	4 cups
Red bell pepper, chopped	1
Yellow onion, chopped	1
Carrots, shredded	2 cups
Sesame oil	1 tbsp.

Chicken Stir-Fry

(all phases ♦ 1 fat)
4 servings

Chicken breasts, chopped	1 lb.
Kale or spinach	1 bag, 9 oz.
Yellow onion, sliced	1
Mushrooms, sliced	1 container, 8–10 oz.
Snap peas	1 bag, 8 oz.
Sesame oil	1 tbsp.

Bring a nonstick pan to medium-high heat, remove from heat, and coat lightly with nonstick cooking spray. Add the protein, cook for 8–10 minutes, adding in 2 tbsp. of sauce for the last 2 minutes, and set aside. In a large wok or sauté pan, add 1 tbsp. of sesame oil, then add the vegetables and sauté 6–8 minutes. Add the protein and heat for another minute. Drain any excess liquid from the vegetables, then add the sauce and remove from heat.

QUICK FIX: Use 2 bags of frozen stir-fry vegetable mix instead of fresh vegetables. Defrost vegetables prior to cooking.

OPTION: If you'd like, you can add fresh cilantro (chopped, 2 tbsp.), fresh basil (chopped, 2 tbsp.), or lemongrass paste to the sauce. (Look for the lemongrass paste in your grocer's refrigerated produce section.)

OPTION: For all of these stir-fries, feel free to mix and match protein and vegetable combinations to fit your taste.

Clinical Pearl: Gluten-Free Soy Sauce Alternatives

Soy sauce is one of the many places that gluten can hide. If you are eliminating gluten from your diet, choose gluten-free soy sauce or tamari sauce, which is often gluten-free. Always check labels for the presence of wheat and other gluten-containing ingredients.

Broiled Fish and Garlic Vegetable Medley

(all phases ◆ 1 fat)
2 servings

For the fish:

Red snapper or other firm whitefish fillets	8 oz.
Kosher salt	1/4 tsp.
Black pepper	1/8 tsp.
Olive oil spray	1/2 tsp.

For the vegetable medley:

Yellow or white onion, chopped	1 cup
Mushrooms, sliced	1 cup
Kale, shredded or chopped, remove stems	4 cups
Olive oil	2 tsp.
Garlic, minced	2 tsp.
Low-sodium vegetable broth*	3–4 tbsp.
Salt	to taste

*OK to use water if you don't have vegetable broth.

Preheat broiler. Season fish with salt and pepper and spray or brush very lightly with olive oil. Arrange fish on a broiler pan coated with nonstick cooking spray and broil 6–8 minutes or until fish flakes easily when tested with a fork. (Fish can also be panfried instead of broiled.) While fish is broiling, prepare vegetable medley. Heat oil in sauté pan. Add garlic and cook for 1 minute. Add vegetables and cook until soft, adding broth as pan heats up to avoid burning vegetables. (Be sure to scrape the side of the pan to add back in the flavorful garlic coating as you are adding broth.) Add salt to taste. Serve over broiled fish.

Asian Lettuce Wraps/Salad

(all phases ◆ 0 fat, 0 dense carbs)
4 servings (approximately
2 cups per serving)

For the chicken:

Extra-lean ground chicken*	16 oz.
Ginger puree	1 tbsp.
Garlic puree	1 tbsp.
Kosher salt	1/2 tsp.
Black pepper	1/4 tsp.
Turmeric	1 tsp.

For the vegetable medley:

Crimini mushrooms, sliced	16 oz.
Broccoli slaw	1 bag, 12 oz.
Cabbage, shredded	10 oz.
Yellow onion, julienned	1 medium
Butter lettuce	1 head

For the sauce:

Soy sauce	1/2 cup
Scallions, chopped	1/4 cup
Ginger, finely chopped	1 tbsp.
Garlic, finely chopped	1 tsp.
Sesame seeds	1 tbsp.
Thai or jalapeño chilies, finely chopped, seeded	1 tsp.
Cilantro, chopped	1 tbsp.
Lime juice	1/2 lime

*For Phase 2, you can use extra-lean ground beef instead.

Bring a nonstick pan to medium heat, remove from heat, and coat lightly with nonstick cooking spray. Add the chicken, ginger and garlic puree, salt, pepper, and turmeric and cook until meat is cooked through, about 6–8 minutes, then place in a bowl and set aside. Wipe the pan clean, then reheat it to medium-high, remove pan from heat, and recoat lightly with nonstick cooking spray. Add all the vegetables and stir-fry for 6–8 minutes, then add the chicken and heat for another 2 minutes and remove from heat. For the butter lettuce, wash, cut off bottom root, and separate the leaves. Mix all sauce ingredients in a small bowl, then scoop some of the meat and veggie mix onto the butter lettuce leaf and spoon sauce over the wraps.

OPTION: Enjoy leftovers as a salad by serving over 2–3 cups of shredded butter lettuce, 1/2 cup shredded carrots, and 1/2 cup water chestnuts. Drizzle with 2 tbsp. sauce.

Fish or Shrimp Tacos   (Phases 2 & 3 ♦ 1 fat, 1½ dense carbs)
                                                              2 servings

For the slaw:

Fat-free sour cream	1/4 cup
Low-fat Greek yogurt	1/4 cup
Cilantro	2 tbsp.
Lime juice	2 tbsp.
Lime zest (optional)	1 tsp.
Kosher salt	1/2 tsp.
Cabbage slaw mix	3 cups

For the fish or shrimp:

Shrimp	12 jumbo
or	
Fish*	8–10 oz.
Chili powder	2 tsp.
Cumin	1 tsp.
Onion powder	1 tsp.
Garlic powder	1 tsp.
Kosher salt	1 tsp.
Black pepper	1/2 tsp.
Olive oil	1 tbsp.
Lime juice	2 tsp. for garnish
Small corn tortillas	4

*You can use mahi mahi, red snapper, or salmon.

For the slaw, mix all ingredients together and refrigerate for 30 minutes. For the seafood, mix all spices together and set aside. Place the seafood of your choice in a sandwich-size ziplock plastic bag and add 1 tbsp. of oil. Add the desired amount of spice mix to the bag and mix, making sure fish or shrimp is coated well with the oil and spices. Let marinade for 1 hour or more—the longer you leave in the marinade, the more intense the flavor will get.

You can either grill the fish/shrimp, roast it under the broiler, or sauté it on your stovetop. If preparing fish on the stovetop, heat your pan on high for

1 minute, remove from heat and coat lightly with nonstick cooking spray, then place fish in the pan and cook for 1 minute. Reduce heat to medium and cook another 4 minutes, then flip and cook for another 3 minutes. (As a rule of thumb, cook fish 1 minute per ounce. So for 8 oz. of fish, cook for 8 minutes—first 5 minutes, then flip and cook another 3 minutes.) If preparing shrimp on the stovetop, heat your pan on high for 1 minute, then remove from heat and coat lightly with nonstick cooking spray. Place shrimp in pan and cook for 1 minute, then reduce heat to medium high and cook for 6–7 more minutes until shrimp is pink. Serve 1/4 fish or shrimp and 1/2 cup slaw in each corn tortilla and eat remainder of slaw as a tasty side salad.

OPTION: Skip the tortillas and serve fish or shrimp over the slaw as a salad.

Chipotle and Turkey Chili

(all phases ◆ 1 dense carb)
6 servings (approximately 2 cups per serving)

For the turkey:

Ground natural turkey	20 oz.
Ground cumin	1 tsp.
Ground garlic	1 tsp.
Chili powder	2 tsp.
Chipotle powder	1/2 tsp.
Ground bay leaf	1/2 tsp.

For the chili:

Yellow onion, diced	2 cups
Carrots, diced	2 cups
Celery, diced	2 cups
Fire-roasted tomatoes	3 cans, 14.5 oz. each
Water	1 cup
Kidney beans	2 cans, 15 oz. each
Vegetable broth	1 carton, 32 oz.
Kosher salt	1 tsp.
Black pepper	1/4 tsp.
Cilantro (optional)	2 tbsp.
Green or red onion, diced (optional)	1/4 cup

Bring a nonstick pan to medium heat, remove the pan from the heat, and coat lightly with nonstick cooking spray. Add turkey, then the spices and bay leaf, and cook until turkey is golden. Add the onion, carrots, and celery and cook until onions get translucent, about 10 minutes. Add the fire-roasted tomatoes and the water and cook for another 10 minutes. Add the kidney beans and vegetable broth, cover, and simmer for 20 minutes. Adjust seasoning with salt and pepper to taste. Top with chopped cilantro or green/red onion if you wish.

QUICK FIX: In a small pot or large microwave-safe bowl, combine a can of low-fat turkey chili with a 14.5 oz. can of fire-roasted tomatoes, 1 tbsp. chili seasoning (from packet), and 1/2 tsp. chipotle powder (optional) and stir well. Simmer uncovered on low to medium heat for 5–10 minutes (stovetop) or heat on high for 2–3 minutes in the microwave loosely covered. Makes 2 servings (1 dense carb).

OPTION: Greens can also be added, such as a bag of fresh or frozen spinach. Defrost frozen spinach and squeeze out the excess water before adding, or add a bag of fresh spinach to the pan during the last 5 minutes of simmering.

OPTION: For Phases 2 and 3, you can use low-fat sour cream or 2% Greek yogurt (2 tbsp.), shredded skim-milk mozzarella or light cheddar (2 tbsp.), or 1/4 sliced avocado (adds 1 fat) as toppings.

Dr. Melina's Tasty Turkey Meat Loaf

(Phases 2 & 3 ♦ 1/2 fat, 1/2 dense carb)
6 servings

For the turkey:

Extra-lean ground turkey	1¼ pounds
Marinara sauce	3/4 cup
Italian-seasoned breadcrumbs	1/2 cup
Parmesan cheese, grated	1/4 cup + 1 tbsp.

For the vegetable medley:

Olive oil	1 tbsp.
Yellow or white onion, finely chopped	1/2 cup
Celery, finely chopped	1/2 cup
Carrots, finely chopped	1/2 cup
Water	2–3 tbsp.

For the meat loaf:

Garlic, minced	1 tsp.
Egg whites	3 large
Basil, dried	1/2 tsp.
Oregano, dried	1/2 tsp.
Salt	1/2 tsp.
Black pepper	1/4 tsp.

Preheat oven to 350 degrees. Coat a pan with the olive oil and sauté onion, celery, and carrot over medium heat until cooked. Add a few tablespoons of water to avoid burning. Cool slightly. Combine ground turkey, 1/2 cup marinara, vegetable mix, and remaining meat loaf ingredients in a large bowl. Shape mixture into an 8 × 4–inch loaf pan coated with cooking spray. Brush remaining 1/4 cup marinara sauce over top of meat loaf and top with remaining tbsp. of Parmesan. Bake for approximately 55 minutes or until cooked through. Let cool 10 minutes before serving.

Italian-Style Tilapia or Cod

(all phases ♦ 1 fat)
4 servings

Tilapia or cod, fresh or frozen*	4 fillets
Olive oil	1½ tbsp.
Garlic, minced	2 cloves or 2 tsp. preminced
Water	1–2 tbsp.
Yellow or white onion, chopped	1 medium
Italian-style diced tomatoes	1 can, 14.5 oz.
Black olives, pitted, sliced	1/2 cup
Parsley, dried	1–2 tsp. or 1 tbsp. fresh
Dry white wine (substitute vegetable broth if you prefer)	1/2 cup

*If you use frozen fish, defrost fully prior to cooking.

In a large frying pan, heat oil and add garlic and onions. Cook until onions soften. Add 1–2 tbsp. water if needed. Stir in tomatoes, olives, parsley, and wine. Simmer for 5 minutes. Place tilapia or cod in sauce and simmer for 5–10 minutes until fish is fully cooked.

Easy Italian Chicken

Boneless, skinless chicken breasts	2 breasts, 4 oz. each
Olive oil	1 tsp.
Garlic powder	1/2 tsp.
Basil, dried	1 tsp.
Salt	to taste
Black pepper	to taste
Marinara sauce	1/2 cup
Reduced-fat shredded mozzarella	1/4 cup

Preheat broiler. Rub top of each chicken breast with 1/2 tsp. olive oil and season with salt, pepper, basil, and garlic powder. Bring a skillet to medium heat, remove from heat, and coat lightly with nonstick cooking spray. Add chicken and cook 6–8 minutes, until cooked through, turning halfway. Remove chicken from skillet and place on baking sheet. Top each cutlet with 1/4 cup marinara sauce and 2 tbsp. cheese. Place under broiler for 1–2 minutes, until cheese is melted. Remove from broiler and serve.

Lemon Shrimp   (all phases ♦ 1 fat)
2 servings

Shrimp, peeled, deveined	12 jumbo
Salt	2 pinches
Black pepper	2 pinches
Olive oil	2 tsp.
White wine*	1/4 cup
Fresh lemon juice	2 tbsp.
Lemon zest	2 tsp.
Capers, drained	1 tbsp.

*OK to use water if you do not have white wine available.

Season shrimp with 1 pinch each salt and pepper. Heat olive oil in a large sauté pan over medium heat. Add shrimp and cook 5 minutes, turning halfway. Remove from pan. Add white wine to pan and heat for 1 minute, scraping up any brown bits on bottom of pan. Reduce heat to low. Add lemon juice, lemon zest, capers, and remaining salt and pepper. Return shrimp to pan and stir well to combine. Remove from heat and serve over preferred whole grain or vegetable.

Rosemary Chicken*   (all phases ♦ 1/2 fat)
                                                    4 servings

Boneless, skinless chicken breast	4 breasts, 3–4 oz. each
Olive oil	2 tsp.
Rosemary, fresh or dried	2 tbsp.
Salt	to taste
Black pepper	to taste

Preheat oven to 450 degrees. Rub each chicken breast with 1/2 tsp. olive oil, 1/2 tbsp. rosemary, and salt and pepper to taste. Bake for 20 minutes or until center is no longer pink and serve.

*Great for leftover salads the next day.

Flank Steak with   (all phases ♦ 1 tsp. sauce = 1 fat)
Chimichurri Sauce   4 servings

Flank steak	1 lb.
Chili powder	2 tsp.
Garlic powder	1 tsp.
Onion powder	1 tsp.
Kosher salt	1/2 tsp.
Black pepper	1/4 tsp.
Olive oil spray	as needed
Chimichurri Sauce	1 tsp.

Mix spices together and rub on both sides of the flank steak. Place in a ziplock bag and refrigerate overnight to get the most flavor into the meat. Preheat broiler, spray both sides of flank steak lightly with olive oil cooking spray, and cook 5–7 minutes per side, then turn off oven and let rest for another minute or two before removing from oven. For outdoor grilling, heat the grill to 500 degrees, spray both sides of flank steak lightly with olive oil cooking spray, then place meat on grate and cook for 5–7 minutes per side. Remove from heat and let it rest for 10 minutes before cutting so that the juices stay in the meat. Top each cooked flank steak with 1 tsp. **Chimichurri Sauce** and serve.

Sweet and Spicy Mango Chicken

(Phases 2 & 3 ◆ 0 fat, 0 dense carbs)
4 servings

Chicken breasts, boneless, skinless	1 lb.

For the marinade:

Mango, frozen*	2 cups
Garlic, smashed	4 cloves
Chili powder	1 tsp.
Turmeric	1 tsp.
Ketchup	1/2 cup
Kosher salt	1 tsp.

*The mango in this dish counts as one serving of fruit.

Puree all the marinade ingredients in a blender. Place chicken in a baking dish and top with marinade. (For better flavor, marinade chicken in refrigerator for at least 30 minutes.) Preheat oven to 450 degrees. Bake for 18–20 minutes until cooked through. For outdoor grilling, use half of the sauce to marinate the chicken in a baking dish. Reserve the rest to brush on while grilling. Marinate chicken breasts for a minimum of 1–2 hours or overnight to get the maximum flavor, then grill over medium heat for about 15–20 minutes.

Vegetarian Lasagna Rolls

(Phases 2 & 3 ◆ 1 dense carb per roll)
6 servings, 2 rolls per serving

Lasagna noodles, cooked and cooled	12

(Use whole-wheat noodles if you can find them)

For the filling:

Garlic, diced	2 cloves
Cottage cheese	3 cups
Basil, fresh	1 bunch
Kosher salt	1 tsp.
Black pepper	1/2 tsp.

For the vegetable medley:

Olive oil	1 tbsp.
Mushrooms, sliced	4 cups
Kale, shredded	1 bunch
or	
Spinach, frozen, defrosted, water squeezed out	2 bags, 1 lb. each

For the topping:

Marinara sauce, jarred	2½ cups
Parmesan cheese	1/2 cup

Preheat oven to 350 degrees. In a food processor, add the garlic, cottage cheese, basil, salt, and pepper, blend until smooth, and set aside. In a sauté pan on high heat, add the oil, then the mushrooms and kale or spinach. Cook for 1 minute and reduce heat to medium-high. Cook until moisture is gone, about 7–8 minutes, and set aside. Lay out your lasagna sheets, spread the cottage cheese mix lengthwise on the noodles, and sprinkle the mushroom and green mix over the cottage cheese. Now roll up all the noodles (you will have 12 rolls). In a 9 × 13–inch pan, add 1 cup of the marinara and spread evenly in dish, then line up the rolls 3 across by 4 rows. Add the remaining marinara to the tops of the noodles and sprinkle with Parmesan cheese. If items are warm to room temperature, bake in a 350 degree oven for 15–18 minutes. If items are from the fridge, cook for 25–35 minutes.

DRESSINGS, DIPS, AND SAUCES

Basic Vinaigrette — (all phases ♦ approximately 1 fat per serving) approximately 5 servings, 2 tbsp. each

Balsamic vinegar	1/4 cup
Water	1/4 cup
Olive oil	2 tbsp.
Dijon mustard	1 tbsp.
Kosher salt	to taste
Black pepper	to taste

Combine all ingredients by stirring with wooden spoon or blending in a blender. Serve or refrigerate. Will last up to 2 weeks in refrigerator.

OPTION: For creamy dressing, combine with 6 oz. plain nonfat Greek yogurt and whisk until smooth. For phases 2 and 3, add 1 tsp. of honey for a less tart dressing.

Asian Vinaigrette

(all phases ♦ approximately 1 fat per serving)
approximately 5 servings, 2 tbsp. each

Rice vinegar	1/4 cup
Water	1/4 cup
Olive oil	2 tbsp.
Ginger	powder1 tsp.
Garlic powder	1 tsp.
Soy sauce	1 tbsp.
Cilantro, chopped	2 tbsp.
Basil, fresh, chopped (optional)	2 tbsp.

Blend all ingredients in a blender and serve or refrigerate. Will last up to 1 week in refrigerator.

OPTION: For creamy dressing, combine with 6 oz. plain nonfat Greek yogurt and whisk until smooth.

Southwest Vinaigrette

(all phases ♦ approximately 1 fat per serving)
approximately 5 servings, 2 tbsp. each

Rice vinegar	1/4 cup
Water	1/4 cup
Olive oil	2 tbsp.
Chili powder	1/2 tsp.
Cumin	1/2 tsp.
Garlic	1/2 tsp.
Onion powder	1/2 tsp.
Green onion, chopped	2 tbsp.
Cilantro, chopped	2 tbsp.
Salt	to taste
Black pepper	to taste

Blend all ingredients in a blender and serve or refrigerate. Will last up to 1 week in refrigerator.

OPTION: For creamy dressing, combine with 6 oz. plain nonfat Greek yogurt and whisk until smooth.

Chimichurri Sauce

(all phases ♦ 1 tsp. = 1 fat)
approximately 24 servings, 1 tsp. each

Apple cider vinegar	3 tbsp.
Olive oil	1/2 cup
Parsley	1 cup packed
Cilantro	1/2 cup packed
Garlic cloves	2–3
Chili flakes	1/4 tsp.
Kosher salt	1 tsp.
Black pepper	1/4 tsp.

Blend all ingredients in a blender until smooth. Spoon onto meat after cooking. Extra sauce may be refrigerated up to a week.

OPTION: Chimichurri sauce is traditionally used with beef, but it is excellent with chicken or fish as well.

Green Goddess-Style Yogurt Dressing/Dip

(all phases ♦ 1/2 fat)
approximately 6 servings, 1/4 cup each

Plain nonfat Greek yogurt	6 oz.
Lemon juice	1 tbsp.
Avocado, peeled, pit removed	1 large
Scallions	4
Basil, fresh	1/4 cup
Italian parsley, fresh	1 tbsp.
Tarragon, fresh	1 tbsp.
Salt	to taste
Black pepper	to taste

Mix all ingredients in food processor or blender until smooth and creamy. Add salt and pepper to taste.

Greek Yogurt Hummus

(all phases ◆ 1/2 dense carb)
approximately 8 servings, 1/4 cup each

Greek yogurt, plain nonfat or low fat yogurt	1/4 cup or 6 oz. individual
Garbanzo beans, drained	1½ cup
Lemon juice	1/4 cup
Garlic, finely chopped	1 tsp.
Cumin	1/4 tsp.
Chili powder	1/4 tsp.
Cayenne pepper (optional)*	1/4 tsp.

*Add the cayenne if you like your food spicy.

Mix all ingredients in a food processor until smooth.

SALADS

QUICK FIX: Use a grocery store rotisserie chicken for any salads requiring chicken (remove the skin) for quicker prep time, or bake several chicken breasts at a time to last you all week.

Crunchy Gazpacho-Style Salad

(all phases ◆ approximately 1 fat)
2 servings

For the shrimp or chicken:

Shrimp or chicken	8 oz.
Chili powder	1 tsp.
Cumin powder	1/2 tsp.
Kosher salt	pinch
Black pepper	pinch

For the gazpacho-style dressing:

Red wine vinegar	3 tbsp.
Lemon juice	1 tbsp.
Olive oil	1 tbsp.

For the salad:

Tomato, diced	1½ cups
Cucumber, English, diced	1 medium
Yellow bell pepper, diced	1 medium

Green onions, chopped small	5
Celery, diced	2 ribs
Baby spinach	4 cups

Season shrimp or chicken with spices, then grill on high heat for 6–8 minutes or until cooked through. If you don't have a grill, then bring a nonstick pan to medium-high heat, remove from heat, and coat lightly with nonstick cooking spray. Add the shrimp or chicken and cook 6–8 minutes or until cooked through. Set aside to cool. Combine ingredients for dressing in a small bowl. Toss all the salad items in a large bowl and add dressing. Top with shrimp or chicken and serve.

QUICK FIX: Use precooked grilled chicken or boiled shrimp and add the chili powder, cumin, salt, and pepper to dressing instead of using it to cook the protein.

Southwest Salmon Cobb Salad

(Phases 2 & 3 ◆ 2 fats, 1/2 dense carb)
1 serving

For the salmon:

Salmon*	3–4 oz.
Chili powder	1 tsp.
Cumin powder	1/2 tsp.
Kosher salt	pinch
Black pepper	pinch

For the salad:

Avocado, diced	1/4
Cherry tomato, sliced	1/4 cup
Black beans	1/4 cup
Mixed greens	2–3 cups
Cilantro, chopped	1 tbsp.
Lime wedge	1–2
Southwest Vinaigrette	2 tbsp.
or	
Low-fat vinaigrette dressing of your choice**	2 tbsp.

*Shrimp, chicken, or beef can also be used for the protein in this dish.

**When shopping for low-fat dressing in the grocery store, look for one that's approximately 50 calories per serving.

Season the fish with the spices and set aside. (Note: This forms a thick, blackened coating on the salmon; if you prefer less spice, cut spice quantities in half.) Bring a nonstick pan to high heat, remove from heat, and coat lightly with nonstick cooking spray. Place the seasoned side of the fish on the pan, cook for 1 minute, reduce heat to medium, cook another 3 minutes, then flip and cook for another 2 minutes and remove from pan. Toss all salad items in a bowl or on a plate.

Mexicali Chicken Salad

(all phases ◆ 1 fat, 1 dense carb)
1 serving

Grilled chicken breast, chopped	2–3 ounces
Romaine lettuce, shredded	3 cups
Black beans	1/2 cup
Avocado, sliced	1/4
Low-fat cheddar cheese, shredded	2 tbsp.
Cilantro, chopped	2 tbsp.
Salsa	1/2 cup

Place lettuce on a plate and top with chicken, black beans, avocado, cheese, cilantro, and salsa as dressing.

OPTION: For Phases 2 and 3, you can use 2 tbsp. of **Southwest Vinaigrette** as dressing (adds 1 fat).

Chopped Chicken Spinach Salad

(all phases ◆ 1 fat, 1/2 dense carb)
1 serving

Grilled chicken, chopped	2–3 ounces
Spinach, chopped	2–3 cups
Carrots, shredded	2 tbsp.
Artichoke hearts, canned, drained	2, cut into quarters
Garbanzo beans, canned, drained	1/4 cup
Cherry tomatoes	8, cut in half
Low-fat mozzarella	2 tbsp.
Basic Vinaigrette	2 tbsp.
or	
Low-fat vinaigrette dressing of your choice	2 tbsp.

Place all ingredients in a medium-size bowl, toss with dressing, and serve.

OPTION: For Phases 2 and 3, half of this salad can be served in 1/2 whole-wheat pita and the rest can be consumed as a side salad.

Steak House Salad   (all phases ♦ 1 fat)
                                                              1 serving

For the steak:

Grilled flank steak	3 oz.
Garlic powder	pinch
Salt	pinch
Black pepper	pinch

For the salad:

Red onion, julienned	1/4
Baby spinach or romaine hearts	2–3 cups
Roma tomato, cut into eighths	1
Blue cheese crumbles	1 tbsp.
Basic Vinaigrette	2 tbsp.
or	
Low-fat vinaigrette dressing of your choice*	2 tbsp.

Season steak with garlic powder, salt, and pepper. Bring a medium sauté pan to medium heat, remove from heat, and coat lightly with nonstick cooking spray. Add onions and sauté until just softened, about 3 minutes. Remove the onions from pan and set aside. Increase heat to medium-high. Add steak and cook for 8–10 minutes, turning halfway. Remove from heat. In a large salad bowl, toss cooked onions, spinach, tomato, and blue cheese with vinaigrette. Slice steak at a 45-degree angle across the grain and layer on top of salad.

QUICK FIX: Use leftover flank steak. If you don't have time to cook the onions, serve them raw as a garnish for the steak or skip them.

Deli Chef Salad   (salad, all phases ♦ 0 fat, 0 dense carbs;
or Pita Pocket   pita pocket, Phases 2 & 3 ♦ 1 fat; 1 dense carb)
                                                              1 serving

Romaine lettuce	2–3 cups
Turkey or chicken, cut into strips or diced	1 oz.
Ham or turkey bacon, cut into strips or diced	1 oz.
Hard-boiled egg, cut into quarters	1

Tomato, diced	1/2
or	
Cherry tomatoes, cut in half	6
Cucumber, sliced or diced	1/2
Blue cheese, crumbled	1 tbsp.
Black olives, sliced (optional)	2 tbsp.
Green onions, chopped (optional)	1–2
Basic Vinaigrette	2 tbsp.
or	
Low-fat vinaigrette dressing of your choice	2 tbsp.

Top lettuce with all ingredients and toss or top with dressing.

OPTION: For Phases 2 and 3, half of this salad can be served in 1/2 whole-wheat pita and the rest can be consumed as a side salad.

Tuna Niçoise Salad

(all phases ♦ 1 fat)
1 serving

For the tuna:

Seared tuna fillet	3 oz.
or	
Water packed-tuna, drained	1/2 of 5 oz. can
Salt	to taste
Black pepper	to taste

For the salad:

Boston (butter) or romaine lettuce	2–3 cups
Haricot vert (thin green beans), steamed	1 cup
Hard-boiled egg, cut into quarters	1
Roma tomato, sliced	1

For the dressing:

Red wine vinegar	1 tbsp.
Dijon mustard	1 tsp.
Olive oil	1 tsp.
Thyme, fresh or dried (optional)	1/2 tsp.

Season tuna with salt and pepper and grill over high heat, or sear in pan coated lightly with nonstick cooking spray, cooking for 1 minute each side. If using canned tuna, drain water and flake with a fork. Top lettuce with haricot vert, hard-boiled egg, and tomato. In small bowl, combine ingredients for dressing and stir. Top salad with grilled or canned tuna and the dressing and serve.

OPTION: For Phases 2 and 3, you can add 1 small red potato (boiled, cut into eighths) and/or 5 Niçoise or Kalamata olives (each cut in half). The potato adds 1 dense carb and the olives add 1 fat.

Gourmet Arugula Chicken Salad

(Phases 2 & 3 ◆ 2 fats)
1 serving

For the chicken salad:

Grilled chicken breast, cut into bite-size pieces	3 oz.
Arugula	2 cups
Edamame, shelled	1/4 cup
Toasted almonds, slivered	1 tbsp.
Parmesan cheese	1 tbsp.

For the dressing:

Lemon	juice of 1/4 lemon + zest of lemon
Olive oil	1 tsp.
Salt	to taste
Black pepper	to taste

Place the arugula, edamame, and almonds in a large bowl. In a smaller bowl, mix the lemon juice, zest, oil, salt, and pepper. Toss with the salad, sprinkle the cheese and chicken on top, and serve.

OPTION: For Phases 2 and 3, serve in 100 calorie wrap or whole-wheat tortilla, or add 1/2 cup faro or barley for an even more satisfying salad.

Mediterranean Chicken or Tuna Salad or Pita Pocket

(salad, all phases ◆ 0 fat, 0 dense carbs; pita pocket, Phases 2 & 3 ◆ 1 fat, 1 dense carb)
1 serving

For the chicken or tuna salad:

Grilled chicken	2–3 oz.
or	
Water-packed tuna, drained	1/2 of 5 oz. can
Spinach, chopped	2–3 cups

Cucumber, peeled, diced	1/2
Cherry tomatoes, cut in half	4
Red onion, diced	1 tbsp.
Kalamata olives, pitted, chopped	1 tbsp.
Lentils	1/3 cup
Feta cheese	1 tbsp.

For the dressing:

Red wine vinegar	1 tbsp.
Olive oil	1 tsp.
Kosher salt	to taste
Black pepper	to taste

Combine spinach, cucumber, tomato, onion, olives, lentils, and feta in medium bowl. In a small bowl, prepare dressing, add to medium bowl, and mix. Top with grilled chicken or tuna and serve.

OPTION: For Phases 2 and 3, omit lentils and serve in 1/2 whole-wheat pita (lightly toasted). Using the whole pita will add 1/2 dense carb.

SIDES

Quinoa Medley

(all phases ◆ 1 dense carb)
4 servings

Quinoa, raw	1/2 cup
Water	1 cup + 2–3 tbsp.
Mushrooms, chopped	1 container, 8 oz.
Yellow or Vidalia onion, diced	1 cup
Garlic, chopped	2 tsp.
Carrots, diced	1½ cups
Salt	1/2 tsp. or to taste

Prepare quinoa per instructions. Stir to make fluffy and set aside. Spray a nonstick pan with nonstick cooking spray. On medium heat, sauté carrots for 3–5 minutes, then add mushrooms and onions and cook for an additional 3–5 minutes or until soft (add 2–3 tbsp. water as needed to prevent vegetables from burning). Add the garlic and cook for another 1–2 minutes. Add quinoa, mix well, cook for another minute, add salt to taste, and serve.

Garlic Vegetable Medley

(all phases ♦ 1 fat)
2 servings

Yellow or Vidalia onion, chopped	1 cup
Mushrooms, sliced	1 cup
Kale, shredded or chopped, remove stems	4 cups
Olive oil	2 tsp.
Low-sodium vegetable broth*	3–4 tbsp.
Garlic, minced	2 tsp.
Salt	1/4 tsp. or to taste

*OK to use water if you don't have vegetable broth.

Heat oil in sauté pan. Add garlic and cook for 1 minute. Add vegetables and cook until soft, adding broth as pan heats up to avoid burning vegetables. Be sure to scrape the side of the pan to add back in the flavorful garlic coating as you are adding broth. Add salt to taste.

Creamed Spinach

(all phases ♦ 0 fat, 0 dense carbs)
2 servings, 1 cup each

Spinach, frozen	1 bag, 16 oz.
Garlic, chopped	1–2 cloves, or 1 tsp. garlic puree
Kosher salt	1/2 tsp.
Black pepper	1/4 tsp.
Plain nonfat Greek yogurt	6 oz.
Parmesan cheese	3 tbsp.

Defrost spinach and squeeze out excess water. In a nonstick pan on medium heat, add the spinach and garlic and season with the salt and pepper. Cook for a few minutes, then add the yogurt and cheese. Cook for another 3–4 minutes until the cheese melts and the yogurt warms up.

Roasted Cauliflower
or Carrots

(all phases ♦ 1/2 fat)
approximately 4 servings

Cauliflower, cut into 1/4 inch pieces	1 head
or	
Carrots, peeled, cut diagonally into pieces	8 large
Olive oil	1 tbsp.
Chili powder	1/4 tsp.

Turmeric	1/4 tsp.
Curry powder	1/4 tsp.
Garlic powder	1/4 tsp.
Kosher salt	1/4 tsp.

Preheat oven to 425 degrees. Place cauliflower or carrots in bowl and toss with oil and spices. Cover a sheet pan with foil, then top with seasoned vegetables. Place in oven and cook for 10 minutes, then flip cauliflower or carrots and cook another 10 minutes. Remove from heat, let cool, and serve.

Cauliflower Mash
(all phases ♦ 1 fat)
2 servings, 1 cup each

Cauliflower	1 head
Garlic powder	1 tsp.
Onion powder	1 tsp.
Salt	1/4 tsp. or to taste
Butter	2 tsp.

This dish can be steamed in the microwave or on the stovetop. If preparing in a microwave, use a steamer that is not made of metal (silicone steamers are microwave-safe). Cook cauliflower until it is soft to the touch. Drain the liquid and set it aside. Then mash the cauliflower with a masher for a chunky style, adding the butter and spices and, if you like, the water to thin the mixture. For a smoother texture, place cauliflower in blender and blend until smooth, adding the oil and spices. If you are making on your stovetop with a pot, add enough water to cover cauliflower and cook until soft. Drain liquid, set it aside, and prepare the dish the same as above.

OPTION: Use the spices from the **Roasted Cauliflower** recipe.

Charred Spicy Green Beans
(all phases ♦ 1/2 fat)
4 servings, 1 cup each

Green beans, cleaned, stems cut off	2 lbs.
Red onion, julienned	1 medium
Roasted green chilies, drained*	1 can, 4 oz.
Olive oil	1 tbsp.
Chili powder	1 tsp.
Cumin	1 tsp.

Kosher salt	1 tsp.
Black pepper	1/4 tsp.
Garlic, minced	3 cloves or 1 tsp. garlic powder
Lemon juice	2 tbsp. (the zest can be added, too)
Almonds, slivered**	1/4 cup

*You can use fresh jalapeño in place of the green chilies if you want. If you like it spicier, use both.

**The slivered almonds are optional for Phases 2 and 3 (adds 1 fat).

In a large bowl, add the green beans, onions, green chilies, olive oil, and spices. Toss together until all green beans are coated. Bring a nonstick sauté pan to high heat, remove pan when hot, and coat lightly with nonstick cooking spray. Add the green bean mix, spreading evenly around the pan. Cook for 1 minute, then toss pan or stir the mix. Continue to do so for 5 minutes, stirring or tossing every minute. Now add the garlic, cook for another minute, remove from heat, and add the lemon juice and, if preferred, the zest.

Spiced Butternut Squash

(all phases ♦ 1 fat, 1 dense carb)
6 servings, approximately
1/2 cup each

For the squash:

| Butternut squash, peeled, seeded, diced into 1 inch pieces* | 1 (3 lbs.) |
| Olive oil | 2 tbsp. |

For the spice mix:

Ground cumin	1½ tsp.
Ground coriander	1 tsp.
Cinnamon	1/4 tsp.
Onion powder	1/4 tsp.
Cayenne pepper	1/8 tsp.
Kosher salt	1/4 tsp.
Black pepper	1/4 tsp.

*You can buy butternut squash already peeled and diced in your grocer's produce section. If you can't, cut the ends off the squash and use a peeler to remove the skin, then cut in half lengthwise, scoop out the seeds, and dice into 1–2 inch pieces.

Preheat the oven to 425 degrees. In a small bowl, combine the spices and set aside. In a large bowl, toss the squash with the olive oil and then add spices and toss until spices are evenly distributed. Spread the squash on a baking sheet in a single layer and roast in the oven for about 30 minutes, until tender and lightly browned, tossing once halfway through. Transfer to a bowl and serve.

OPTION: This recipe produces a lot of squash, but it's so delicious you will probably want it for leftovers. If you would rather cook less or are using bags of precut squash, cut spices and oil in half and use 1½ pounds of squash instead.

Zucchini Parmesan   (all phases ♦ 1 fat)
                                                          4 servings

For the zucchini:

Zucchini, quartered lengthwise	4
Olive oil	1 tbsp.

For the Parmesan topping:

Parmesan cheese, grated	1/2 cup
Thyme, dried	1/2 tsp.
Basil, dried	1/2 tsp.
Oregano, dried	1/2 tsp.
Salt	1/4 tsp. or to taste

Preheat oven to 350 degrees. Combine Parmesan cheese and herbs in a small bowl and set aside. Lightly coat baking sheet with nonstick cooking spray. Toss zucchini with olive oil and place on baking sheet. Top evenly with Parmesan blend. Bake at 350 degrees for 10–13 minutes, until soft.

OPTION: Broil for additional 2–3 minutes until top is golden brown.

Roasted Brussels Sprouts   (all phases ♦ 1 fat)
                                                          4 servings

Brussels sprouts, cleaned, dried, halved*	1 lb.
Garlic, minced	3 cloves
Kosher salt	1/4 tsp.
Black pepper	1/4 tsp.
Olive oil	4 tsp.
Balsamic vinegar	2 tbsp.

*This recipe also works well with broccoli in place of the Brussels sprouts. Just skip the balsamic vinegar and make sure broccoli is very dry before tossing with oil, garlic, salt, and pepper.

Preheat oven to 400 degrees. In a large mixing bowl, combine Brussels sprouts, garlic, salt, and pepper. Add olive oil to coat well. Pour Brussels sprouts mixture onto a large, shallow sheet or roasting pan and drizzle with balsamic vinegar. Toss again gently to spread the Brussels sprouts evenly on the pan. Roast in the oven for 25–30 minutes, until sprouts are slightly brown and fork tender, stirring once or twice halfway through cooking.

SOUPS AND SLOW COOKER MEALS

Dr. Melina's Doctor on Demand Pureed Vegetable Soup

(all phases ♦ 0 fat, 0 dense carbs)
approximately 10 servings, 1 cup each

Have this soup as an appetizer to help you feel full faster, or enjoy a cup between meals for a super satisfying, light snack. Many people find the pureed version more delicious and filling, but feel free to enjoy it chunky-style if you prefer.

For the vegetable medley:

Leeks, chopped	3 large
Garlic, minced	3 cloves
Cauliflower, chopped	1 head
Carrots, chopped	1 cup
Celery, chopped	1 cup
Olive oil	1 tbsp.
Water	1/4 cup
Kosher salt	pinch, + to taste

For the stock:

Chicken broth	2 quarts
Thyme	1–2 tsp.
Black pepper	1/4 tsp.
Bay leaf	1
Spinach, fresh	1 bag, 10–14 oz.

Heat a large stockpot on high heat and add the olive oil. When oil is hot, add the leeks, garlic, water, and a pinch of salt and cook for 5 minutes until soft, stirring frequently. Add the cauliflower, carrots, and celery and cook for 5 minutes. When vegetables are beginning to soften, add the chicken broth, thyme, pepper, and bay leaf and bring to a boil, then reduce heat and simmer on medium-low heat for 20 minutes. Add the bag of spinach, simmer for an additional 5 minutes, and remove from heat. Use an immersion stick blender or regular blender to puree soup until smooth. Salt to taste.

Minestrone Soup

(all phases ◆ 1 dense carb)
6 servings, approximately 1½ cups each

Tomatoes, diced	2 cans, 14.5 oz. each
Tomato paste	2 tbsp.
Vegetable stock	5 cups
Water	2 cups
Carrots, diced	1 cup
Celery, diced	1¼ cup
White onion, diced	1½ cup
Garlic, minced	4–5 cloves
Oregano	4 sprigs or 1 tsp. dried
Rosemary	1 sprig or 1/2 teaspoon dried
Thyme	4 sprigs or 1/2 teaspoon dried
Bay leaves	2
Kidney beans, drained, rinsed	2 cans, 15 oz. each
Zucchini, diced	1½ cups
Yellow squash, diced	1½ cups
Green beans, cut into 2 inch pieces	1 cup
Spinach, frozen, chopped	1 bag, 16 oz.
Kosher salt	to taste
Black pepper	to taste

Add the diced tomatoes, tomato paste, vegetable stock, water, carrots, celery, onions, garlic, oregano, rosemary, thyme, and bay leaves to a slow cooker. Cook on low heat 5–6 hours or high 3–4 hours. Then add the kidney beans, squash, zucchini, spinach, and green beans and cook on high heat for an additional 20–25 minutes. Add salt and pepper to taste.

Pork Loin "Adobo" Style

(all phases ◆ 0 fat, 0 dense carbs)
4 servings

Pork loin, cubed	1 lb.
Low-sodium soy sauce*	1/4 cup
Apple cider vinegar	1/4 cup
Water	1/3 cup
Yellow onion, diced	1 medium
Garlic, smashed	4 cloves
Chipotle pepper, chopped	1
Black pepper	1/4 tsp.
Bay leaf	2

Place all ingredients in slow cooker and cook on low heat for 6–8 hours.

Braised Chard and Vegetables

(all phases ◆ 0 fat, 0 dense carbs)
approximately 6 servings

Swiss chard, chopped	1 bunch
Zucchini, diced medium	1 large
Eggplant, diced medium	1 large
Mushrooms, sliced	1 container, 8 oz.
Yellow onion, diced medium	1 large
Garlic, chopped	1 tbsp.
Basil, fresh, chopped	1/4 cup
Chili powder	1 tsp.
Cherry tomatoes	1 pint
White wine	1/4 cup
Rosemary	2 sprigs
Thyme, fresh	4 sprigs
Kosher salt	1 tsp.
Black pepper	1/2 tsp.

Place all ingredients except the herbs in slow cooker and stir to mix. Add the rosemary and thyme on top and cook on high for 2 hours. Once cooked, adjust salt and pepper.

OPTION: Top with 1 tbsp. fresh Parmesan cheese.

SANDWICHES AND WRAPS

Herbed Tuna Melt   (Phases 2 & 3 ◆ 1 fat, 1 dense carb)
4 servings

Water-packed tuna, drained	2 cans, 6 oz. each
Low-fat mayonnaise	4 tbsp.
Dijon mustard	2 tbsp.
Parsley, flat leaf, chopped	3 tbsp.
Tarragon, fresh	2 tbsp. or 2 tsp. dried
Green onion, thinly sliced	1
Lemon zest	1 lemon
Lemon juice	2 tsp.
Black pepper	1/8 tsp.
Kosher salt	1 tsp.
Whole-grain bread	4 slices
Low-fat cheddar cheese, shredded	1/2 cup
Tomato, sliced	1

In a bowl, mix together the mayo, mustard, parsley, tarragon, green onion, lemon juice and zest, pepper, and salt. Fold in the tuna and mix evenly. Place bread in toaster and toast to desired crunch. As soon as the toast pops up, place one piece of cheese on the bread to melt, then add the tomato slices and top with tuna.

Grilled Chicken TBLT Wrap   (Phases 2 & 3 ◆ 1 fat, 1 dense carb)
1 serving

Boneless, skinless chicken breast	2–3 oz.
Turkey bacon, crumbled	1 slice
Salt	pinch
Black pepper	pinch
Garlic powder	pinch
Romaine lettuce, shredded	1 cup
Grape tomatoes, halved	1/2 cup
Basic Vinaigrette	2 tbsp.
or	
Low-fat vinaigrette dressing of your choice	2 tbsp.
Whole-wheat wrap (100 calories or less)	1

Preheat grill or broiler. Cook turkey bacon as directed. Season chicken with salt, pepper, and garlic powder. Grill or broil chicken 8–10 minutes or until chicken reaches an internal temperature of 165 degrees), turning halfway. Remove from heat and slice. In medium bowl, toss lettuce, tomatoes, chicken, and crumbled turkey bacon with vinaigrette. Pour into whole-wheat wrap or 1/2 whole-wheat pita and serve. If you have extra filling, eat as a side salad.

QUICK FIX: Use store-bought rotisserie chicken (remove skin) in place of chicken breasts.

Turkey Hummus Wrap   (Phases 2 & 3 ♦ 1 dense carb)
                                                              1 serving

Whole-wheat tortilla or 100 calorie wrap	1
Greek Yogurt Hummus	2–3 tbsp.
Turkey, sliced	3 oz.
Cucumber, sliced*	1/2
Red bell pepper, sliced or diced	1/2 cup
Romaine lettuce, chopped	1 cup

*Eat the other half of the cucumber on the side.

Spread hummus on tortilla or wrap, top with turkey and vegetables, and roll into wrap. Use any extra vegetables that don't fit into your wrap as a side salad. If using store-bought hummus, also count as 1 fat.

BBQ Chicken Pita Pizza   (Phases 2 & 3 ♦ 1½ dense carbs)
                                                              1 serving

Whole-wheat pita	1
BBQ sauce	2–3 tbsp.
Chicken breast, diced	3 oz.
Red onion, julienned	2 tbsps.
Low-fat mozzarella	1/4 cup

Preheat oven to 400 degrees. Top whole-wheat pita with BBQ sauce, chicken breast, 2 tbsp. julienned onions, and low-fat mozzarella. Place on cookie sheet and bake about 10 minutes, until cheese is melted.

DESSERTS

Baked Apple or Pear   (all phases ♦ 0 fat, 0 dense carbs)
                                                                  1 serving

Fuji apple or Bartlett pear, halved,
    seeds and stem removed   1
Cinnamon*   1 tsp.

*Apple pie spice or pumpkin pie spice can be used in place of cinnamon. Ginger can be used in place of or in addition to cinnamon for the baked pear.

Preheat oven to 350 degrees. Sprinkle each half with 1/2 tsp. cinnamon and cook apple or pear halves for 20–25 minutes (20 minutes will give you fruit that is soft but still a little firm).

QUICK FIX: Prepare in microwave. Heat in covered glass dish on high for 3–5 minutes until soft to touch (total time depends on the size of the fruit).

OPTION: Bake an extra apple or pear to use in your smoothie or parfait the next day!

Baked Apple or Pear Crumble   (Flex Block)
                                                                  2 servings

Fuji apple or Bartlett pear, halved,
    seeds and stem removed   1
Oats   1/4 cup
Brown sugar   1 tbsp.
Flour or oat flour   1 tbsp.
Cinnamon   1/2 tsp.
Nutmeg   1/8 tsp.
Almonds or pecans, chopped   1 tbsp.
Butter   1 tbsp.

Preheat oven to 350 degrees. In a bowl, combine the oats, brown sugar, flour, cinnamon, nutmeg, and nuts. Blend the butter into the dry ingredients using a fork or your fingers, until the mixture resembles coarse crumbs. Place the topping on the apple or pear halves and bake for 20 minutes.

Sweet Ricotta   (all phases ◆ 0 fat, 0 dense carbs)
                                                            1 serving

| Low-fat ricotta cheese | 1/4 cup |
| Stevia | 1 packet |

Combine and serve.

OPTION: Top with 1/2 cup fresh berries or 1 tbsp. chopped nuts.

Cinnamon Ricotta   (dip, all phases ◆ 0 fats, 0 dense carbs;
Dip/Crunch   crunch, Phases 2 & 3 ◆ 1 fat)
                                                            1 serving

Low-fat ricotta cheese	2 tbsp.
Stevia	1/2 packet
Cinnamon	1/8 tsp.

Combine all ingredients in a small bowl and serve as dip with fruit.

OPTION: For Phases 2 and 3, double the recipe and top with 1 tbsp. chopped almonds for a delicious dessert.

Honey Ricotta Crunch   (Phases 2 & 3 ◆ 1 fat)
                                                            1 serving

Low-fat ricotta cheese	1/4 cup
Honey	1–2 tsp. (to desired sweetness)
Almonds or peanuts, crushed	1 tbsp.

Combine ricotta and honey in a small bowl and mix well. Place nuts in a small ziplock plastic bag and crush. Top honey ricotta with crushed nuts and serve.

Chocolate Strawberry   (Flex Block)
Dessert Parfait   1 serving

Low-sugar vanilla yogurt	1/2 cup
Mini chocolate chips	2 tsp.
Strawberries	4 sliced
or	
Raspberries	1/2 cup

Mix yogurt with chocolate chips, top with berries, and serve.

OPTION: You can substitute 1 tbsp. slivered almonds for the berries.

Coconut Mango Dessert Parfait   (Phases 2 & 3 ♦ 1 fat)
                                                        1 serving

Nonfat vanilla yogurt	1/2 cup
Turmeric	dash
Mango, sliced	1/2 cup
Toasted coconut	1 tbsp.

Mix turmeric with yogurt and top with sliced mango and toasted coconut.

Chocolate Dipped Fruit   (Flex Block)
                                                       2 servings

Semisweet or dark chocolate chips	3 tbsp.
Banana, sliced	1
or	
Strawberries	8–10

Heat chocolate chips in small glass bowl in microwave until melted, approximately 1 minute. Serve immediately as dip for fruit, or dip fruit in chocolate, place on wax paper, refrigerate for 15–20 minutes until chocolate is firm, and serve.

Bibliography

Chapter 1: The CleanStart Plan

Abargouei AS, Janghorbani M, Salehi-Marzijarani M, Esmaillzadeh A. "Effect of Dairy Consumption on Weight and Body Composition in Adults: A Systematic Review and Meta-Analysis of Randomized Controlled Clinical Trials." *International Journal of Obesity* 2012 Dec;36(12):1485–93.
http://www.ncbi.nlm.nih.gov/pubmed/22249225

Casazza K, et al. "Myths, Presumptions, and Facts about Obesity." *New England Journal of Medicine* 2013 Jan 31;368(5):446–54.
http://www.ncbi.nlm.nih.gov/pmc/articles/PMC3606061/

"Celiac Disease Symptoms." Celiac Disease Foundation.
http://celiac.org/celiac-disease/symptoms/

"Dietary Reference Intakes for Energy, Carbohydrate, Fiber, Fat, Fatty Acids, Cholesterol, Protein, and Amino Acids." Institute of Medicine.
http://www.iom.edu/Reports/2002/Dietary-Reference-Intakes-for
-Energy-Carbohydrate-Fiber-Fat-Fatty-Acids-Cholesterol-Protein
-and-Amino-Acids.aspx

Fuhrman J, Sarter B, Glaser D, Acocella S. "Changing Perceptions of Hunger on a High Nutrient Density Diet." *Nutrition Journal* 2010 Nov 7;9:51.
http://www.ncbi.nlm.nih.gov/pubmed/21054899

Hong HR, Jeong JO, Kong JY, Lee SH, Yang SH, Ha CD, Kang HS. "Effect of Walking Exercise on Abdominal Fat, Insulin Resistance, and Serum Cytokines in Obese Women." *Journal of Exercise Nutrition and Biochemistry* 2014 Sep;18(3):277–85.
http://www.ncbi.nlm.nih.gov/pubmed/25566464

Karalus M, Clark M, Greaves KA, Thomas W, Vickers Z, Kuyama M, Slavin J. "Fermentable Fibers Do Not Affect Satiety or Food Intake

by Women Who Do Not Practice Restrained Eating." *Journal of the Academy of Nutrition and Dietetics* 2012 Sep;112(9):1356–62.
http://www.ncbi.nlm.nih.gov/pubmed/22771185

"Low-Calorie Sweeteners." American Diabetes Association.
http://www.diabetes.org/food-and-fitness/food/what-can-i-eat/
understanding-carbohydrates/artificial-sweeteners/

Mattes RD, Kris-Etherton PM, Foster GD. "Impact of Peanuts and Tree Nuts on Body Weight and Healthy Weight Loss in Adults." *Journal of Nutrition* 2008 Sep;138(9):1741S–5S.
http://www.ncbi.nlm.nih.gov/pubmed/18716179

Nackers LM, Ross KM, Perri MG. "The Association between Rate of Initial Weight Loss and Long-Term Success in Obesity Treatment: Does Slow and Steady Win the Race?" *International Journal of Behavioral Medicine* 2010 Sep;17(3):161–7.
http://www.ncbi.nlm.nih.gov/pubmed/20443094

"Omega-3 Fatty Acids." National Center for Complementary and Alternative Medicine.
http://nccam.nih.gov/health/omega3

Oppezzo M, Schwartz DL. "Give Your Ideas Some Legs: The Positive Effect of Walking on Creative Thinking." *Journal of Experimental Psychology, Learning, Memory, and Cognition* 2014 Jul;40(4):1142–52.
http://www.ncbi.nlm.nih.gov/pubmed/24749966

Pal S, Radavelli-Bagatini S. "The Effects of Whey Protein on Cardio-metabolic Risk Factors." *Obesity Reviews* 2013 Apr;14(4):324–43.
http://www.ncbi.nlm.nih.gov/pubmed/23167434

"Protein." Centers for Disease Control and Prevention.
http://www.cdc.gov/nutrition/everyone/basics/protein.html

"Publications by Barbara Rolls." The Laboratory for the Study of Human Ingestive Behavior at the Pennsylvania State University.
http://nutrition.psu.edu/foodlab/publications

Rebello CJ, Greenway FL, Finley JW. "A Review of the Nutritional Value of Legumes and Their Effects on Obesity and Its Related Co-Morbidities." *Obesity Reviews* 2014 May;15(5):392–407.
http://www.ncbi.nlm.nih.gov/pubmed/24433379

"Thyroid Disease." American Thyroid Association.
http://www.thyroid.org/media-main/about-hypothyroidism/

"What is Celiac Disease?" Celiac Disease Foundation.
http://celiac.org/celiac-disease/what-is-celiac-disease/

Chapter 2: The Customize Your Carbs Plan

"All About Insulin Resistance." American Diabetes Association.
http://professional.diabetes.org/admin/UserFiles/file/Reducing%20
Cardiometabolic%20Risk_%20Patient%20Education%20Toolkit/
English/ADA%20CMR%20Toolkit_2Insulin.pdf

"Am I at Risk for Type-2 Diabetes? Taking Steps to Lower Your Risk of
Getting Diabetes." US Department of Health and Human Services
National Diabetes Information Clearinghouse.
http://diabetes.niddk.nih.gov/dm/pubs/riskfortype2/index.aspx

Anton SD, Martin CK, Han H, Coulon S, Cefalu WT, Geiselman P,
Williamson DA. "Effects of Stevia, Aspartame, and Sucrose on
Food Intake, Satiety, and Postprandial Glucose and Insulin Levels."
Appetite 2010 Aug;55(1):37–43.
http://www.ncbi.nlm.nih.gov/pubmed/20303371

Baburao A, Souza GD. "Insulin Resistance in Moderate to Severe
Obstructive Sleep Apnea in Nondiabetics and Its Response to
Continuous Positive Airway Pressure Treatment." *North American
Journal of Medical Sciences* 2014 Oct;6(10):500–4.
http://www.ncbi.nlm.nih.gov/pubmed/25489561

"Diagnosis of Diabetes and Pre-Diabetes." US Department of Health and
Human Services National Diabetes Information Clearinghouse.
http://diabetes.niddk.nih.gov/dm/pubs/diagnosis/

"Insulin Resistance and Prediabetes." US Department of Health and
Human Services National Diabetes Information Clearinghouse.
http://diabetes.niddk.nih.gov/dm/pubs/insulinresistance/

"Magnesium." National Institutes of Health Office of Dietary
Supplements.
http://ods.od.nih.gov/factsheets/Magnesium-Consumer/#h5

Miller PE, Perez V. "Low-Calorie Sweeteners and Body Weight Composition: A Meta-Analysis of Randomized Controlled Clinical Trials and Prospective Cohort Studies." *American Journal of Clinical Nutrition* 2014 Sep;100(3):765–77.
http://www.ncbi.nlm.nih.gov/pubmed/24944060

O'Connor LM, Lentjes MA, Luben RN, Khaw KT, Wareham NJ, Forouhi NG. "Dietary Dairy Product Intake and Incident Type 2 Diabetes: A Prospective Study Using Dietary Data from a 7-Day Food Diary." *Diabetologia* 2014 May;57(5):909–17.
http://www.ncbi.nlm.nih.gov/pubmed/24510203

"Small Steps. Big Rewards. Prevent Type 2 Diabetes Campaign." National Diabetes Education Program.
http://ndep.nih.gov/partners-community-organization/campaigns/SmallStepsBigRewards.aspx

"U.S. Adult Consumption of Added Sugars Increased by More Than 30% Over Three Decades." Obesity Society.
http://www.obesity.org/news-center/us-adult-consumption-of-added-sugars-increased-by-more-than-30-over-three-decades.htm

Chapter 3: The Cycle for Success Plan

Eshghinia S, Mohammadzadeh F. "The Effects of Modified Alternate-Day Fasting Diet on Weight Loss and CAD Risk Factors in Overweight and Obese Women." *Journal of Diabetes and Metabolic Disorders* 2013 Jan 9;12(1):4.
http://www.ncbi.nlm.nih.gov/pubmed/23497604

"Thinking About the Long-Term Impact of Your Food Choices May Help Control Food Cravings." Obesity Society.
http://www.obesity.org/news-center/thinking-about-the-long-term-impact-of-your-food-choices-may-help-control-food-cravings.htm

Varady KA et al. "Alternate Day Fasting for Weight Loss in Normal Weight and Overweight Subjects: A Randomized Controlled Trial." *Nutrition Journal* 2013, 12:146.
http://www.nutritionj.com/content/12/1/146

Chapter 4: Fire Up Your Future with Goals That Deliver

"Body Mass Index Table." National Heart, Lung, and Blood Institute.
   http://www.nhlbi.nih.gov/health/educational/lose_wt/BMI/bmi
   _tbl.htm

"Calculate Your Body Mass Index." National Heart, Lung, and Blood
   Institute.
   http://www.nhlbi.nih.gov/health/educational/lose_wt/BMI/bmicalc
   .htm

"Diabetes Prevention Program." US Department of Health and Human
   Services National Diabetes Information Clearinghouse.
   http://diabetes.niddk.nih.gov/dm/pubs/preventionprogram/

"Overweight and Obesity Statistics." National Institute of Diabetes and
   Digestive and Kidney Diseases.
   http://win.niddk.nih.gov/statistics/

Chapter 6: Get Moving: Exercise and Activity Strategies That Really Work

"Blood Glucose Control and Exercise." American Diabetes Association.
   http://www.diabetes.org/food-and-fitness/fitness/get-started
   -safely/blood-glucose-control-and-exercise.html

"Exercise or Physical Activity FastStats." Centers for Disease Control and
   Prevention.
   http://www.cdc.gov/nchs/fastats/exercise.htm

Holmstrup ME, Fairchild TJ, Keslacy S, Weinstock RS, Kanaley JA.
   "Satiety, but Not Total PYY, Is Increased with Continuous and
   Intermittent Exercise." *Obesity* 2013 Oct;21(10):2014–20.
   http://www.ncbi.nlm.nih.gov/pubmed/23418154

"How Much Physical Activity Do Adults Need?" Centers for Disease
   Control and Prevention.
   http://www.cdc.gov/physicalactivity/everyone/guidelines/adults
   .html

Levine JA, Vander Weg MW, Hill JO, Klesges RC, "Non-Exercise
   Activity Thermogenesis: The Crouching Tiger Hidden Dragon of

Societal Weight Gain." *Arteriosclerosis, Thrombosis, and Vascular Biology* 2006; 26: 729–36.
http://atvb.ahajournals.org/content/26/4/729.full

Levine, James A. *Get Up: Why Your Chair is Killing You and What You Can Do About It.* New York: Palgrave Macmillan, 2014.
http://www.amazon.com/Get-Up-Chair-Killing-About/dp/1137278994

Mitranun W, Deerochanawong C, Tanaka H, Suksom D. "Continuous vs. Interval Training on Glycemic Control and Macro- and Microvascular Reactivity in Type 2 Diabetic Patients." *Scandinavian Journal of Medicine & Science in Sports* 2014 Apr;24(2):e69–76.
http://www.ncbi.nlm.nih.gov/pubmed/24102912

Sjögren P, Fisher R, Kallings L, Svenson U, Roos G, Hellénius ML. "Stand Up for Health—Avoiding Sedentary Behaviour Might Lengthen Your Telomeres: Secondary Outcome from a Physical Activity RCT in Older People." *British Journal of Sports Medicine* 2014 Oct;48(19):1407–9.
http://www.ncbi.nlm.nih.gov/pubmed/25185586

"The 'NEAT Defect' in Human Obesity: The Role of Nonexercise Activity Thermogenesis." *Mayo Clinic Endocrinology Update* 2007;2(1):1-2.
http://www.mayoclinic.org/documents/mc5810-0307-pdf/doc -20079082

"The N.E.A.T. Way to Exercise." American Council on Exercise.
http://www.acefitness.org/acefit/healthy-living-article/60/3757/ the-n-e-a-t-way-to-exercise/

Chapter 7: Get Your Head in the Game: Understanding the Psychological Side of Weight Loss

"Binge Eating Disorder Fact Sheet." Office on Women's Health, US Department of Health and Human Services.
http://www.womenshealth.gov/publications/our-publications/ fact-sheet/binge-eating-disorder.html

Bodnar LM, Wisner KL. "Nutrition and Depression: Implications for Improving Mental Health Among Childbearing-Aged Women." *Biological Psychiatry* 2005 Nov 1;58(9):679–85.
http://www.ncbi.nlm.nih.gov/pubmed/16040007

Brinkworth GD, Buckley JD, Noakes M, Clifton PM, Wilson CJ. "Long-Term Effects of a Very Low-Carbohydrate Diet and a Low-Fat Diet on Mood and Cognitive Function." *Archives of Internal Medicine* 2009 Nov 9;169(20):1873–80.
http://www.ncbi.nlm.nih.gov/pubmed/19901139

"Depression Fact Sheet." Office on Women's Health, US Department of Health and Human Services.
http://www.womenshealth.gov/publications/our-publications/fact-sheet/depression.html

"Feeding and Eating Disorders." American Psychiatric Association.
http://www.dsm5.org/documents/eating%20disorders%20fact%20sheet.pdf

Flint AJ, Gearhardt AN, Corbin WR, Brownell KD, Field AE, Rimm EB. "Food-Addiction Scale Measurement in 2 Cohorts of Middle-Aged and Older Women." *American Journal of Clinical Nutrition* 2014 Mar;99(3):578–86.
http://www.ncbi.nlm.nih.gov/pubmed/24452236

Geller SE, Studee L. "Botanical and Dietary Supplements for Mood and Anxiety in Menopausal Women." *Menopause* 2007 May-Jun;14 (3 Pt 1):541–9.
http://www.ncbi.nlm.nih.gov/pubmed/17194961

Herman BK, Safikhani S, Hengerer D, Atkins N, Kim A, Cassidy D, Babcock T, Agus S, Lenderking WR. "The Patient Experience with DSM-5-Defined Binge Eating Disorder: Characteristics, Barriers to Treatment, and Implications for Primary Care Physicians." *Postgraduate Medicine* 2014 Sep;126(5):52–63.
http://www.ncbi.nlm.nih.gov/pubmed/25295650

Kessler, David A. *The End of Overeating: Taking Control of the Insatiable American Appetite.* Emmaus, PA: Rodale Books, 2010.
http://www.amazon.com/End-Overeating-Insatiable-American-Appetite/dp/1605294578/ref=tmm_pap_swatch_0?_encoding=UTF8&sr=8-1&qid=1415813622

"New in the DSM-5: Binge Eating Disorder." National Eating Disorders Association.
http://www.nationaleatingdisorders.org/new-dsm-5-binge-eating-disorder

"Patient Health Questionnaire Screeners: Overview." Pfizer Inc.
http://www.phqscreeners.com/overview.aspx

"Patient Health Questionnaire Screeners: Scoring." Pfizer Inc.
http://www.phqscreeners.com/instructions/instructions.pdf

"Yale Food Addiction Scale." Yale University Rudd Center for Food Policy & Obesity.
http://www.yaleruddcenter.org/resources/upload/docs/what/addiction/foodaddictionscale09.pdf

Chapter 8: Create an Environment That Supports Success

"Beating Mindless Eating." Cornell University Food and Brand Lab.
http://www.foodpsychology.cornell.edu/research/beating-mindless-eating.html

Christakis NA, Fowler JH. "The Spread of Obesity in a Large Social Network over 32 Years." *New England Journal of Medicine* 2007 Jul 26;357(4):370–9.
http://www.ncbi.nlm.nih.gov/pubmed/17652652

Nikolaou CK, Hankey CR, and Lean MEJ. "Preventing Weight Gain with Calorie Labeling." *Obesity* 2014 November;22(11):2277–2283.
http://onlinelibrary.wiley.com/doi/10.1002/oby.20885/abstract

Wansink B, Payne CR, Shimizu M. "The 100-Calorie Semi-Solution: Sub-Packaging Most Reduces Intake among the Heaviest." *Obesity* 2011 May;19(5):1098–100.
http://www.ncbi.nlm.nih.gov/pubmed/21233814

Wansink, Brian. *Mindless Eating: Why We Eat More Than We Think*. New York: Bantam Paperback, 2007.

http://www.amazon.com/Mindless-Eating-More-Than-Think/
dp/0553384481/ref=tmm_pap_swatch_0?_encoding
=UTF8&sr=&qid

Wansink, Brian. *Slim by Design: Mindless Eating Solutions for Everyday Life*. New York: William Morrow, 2014.

http://www.amazon.com/Slim-Design-Mindless-Solutions-Everyday/
dp/0062136526/ref=sr_1_1?ie=UTF8&qid=1415811946&sr=8-1&
keywords=Brian+Wansink

Chapter 9: Eating in the Real World

Bes-Rastrollo M, et al. "A Prospective Study of Eating Away-from-Home Meals and Weight Gain in a Mediterranean Population: The SUN (Seguimiento Universidad de Navarra) Cohort." *Public Health Nutrition* 2010 Sep;13(9):1356–63.

http://www.ncbi.nlm.nih.gov/pubmed/19954575

Flood-Obbagy JE, Rolls BJ. "The Effect of Fruit in Different Forms on Energy Intake and Satiety at a Meal." *Appetite* 2009 Apr; 52(2):416–22.

http://www.ncbi.nlm.nih.gov/pubmed/19110020

Nguyen BT, Powell LM. "The Impact of Restaurant Consumption among US Adults: Effects on Energy and Nutrient Intakes." *Public Health Nutrition* 2014 Nov;17(11):2445–52.

http://www.ncbi.nlm.nih.gov/pubmed/25076113

Orsama AL, Mattila E, Ermes M, van Gils M, Wansink B, Korhonen I. "Weight Rhythms: Weight Increases during Weekends and Decreases during Weekdays." *Obesity Facts* 2014;7(1):36–47.

http://www.ncbi.nlm.nih.gov/pubmed/24504358

Chapter 10: Maintaining Your Weight Loss: Seven Steps to Lifelong Success

Azadbakht L, Mirmiran P, Esmaillzadeh A, Azizi F. "Better Dietary Adherence and Weight Maintenance Achieved by a

Long-Term Moderate-Fat Diet." *British Journal of Nutrition* 2007 Feb;97(2):399–404.

http://www.ncbi.nlm.nih.gov/pubmed/17298711

Layman DK, Evans EM, Erickson D, Seyler J, Weber J, Bagshaw D, Griel A, Psota T, Kris-Etherton P. "A Moderate-Protein Diet Produces Sustained Weight Loss and Long-Term Changes in Body Composition and Blood Lipids in Obese Adults." *Journal of Nutrition* 2009 Mar;139(3):514–21.

http://www.ncbi.nlm.nih.gov/pubmed/19158228

"Low-Energy-Dense Foods and Weight Management: Cutting Calories While Controlling Hunger." Centers for Disease Control and Prevention.

http://www.cdc.gov/nccdphp/dnpa/nutrition/pdf/r2p_energy
     _density.pdf

Raynor HA, Van Walleghen EL, Bachman JL, Looney SM, Phelan S, Wing RR. "Dietary Energy Density and Successful Weight Loss Maintenance." *Eating Behaviors* 2011 Apr;12(2):119–25.

http://www.ncbi.nlm.nih.gov/pubmed/21385641

Sumithran P, Proietto J. "The Defence [sic] of Body Weight: A Physiological Basis for Weight Regain after Weight Loss." *Clinical Science* 2013 Feb;124(4):231–41.

http://www.ncbi.nlm.nih.gov/pubmed/23126426

Teixeira PJ, Silva MN, Coutinho SR, Palmeira AL, Mata J, Vieira PN, Carraça EV, Santos TC, Sardinha LB. "Mediators of Weight Loss and Weight Loss Maintenance in Middle-Aged Women." *Obesity* 2010 Apr;18(4):725–35.

http://www.ncbi.nlm.nih.gov/pubmed/19696752